Nutrition and patients

A doctor's responsibility

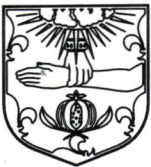

**Report of a working party of the
ROYAL COLLEGE OF PHYSICIANS**

2002

Royal College of Physicians of London
11 St Andrews Place, London NW1 4LE
Registered Charity No 210508

Copyright © 2002 Royal College of Physicians of London
ISBN 1 86016 164 2

Text editing and layout by the Publications Department
of the Royal College of Physicians

Cover design by Merriton Sharp

Cover illustration from an eighteenth century caricature, origin unknown

Typeset by Dan-Set Graphics, Telford, Shropshire

Printed in Great Britain by Sarum ColourView Group, Salisbury, Wiltshire

Contents

Foreword

Nutrition is now high on the public agenda, but unfortunately it is often overlooked by doctors. Under- and overnutrition are, however, clinically important. Obesity has become so prevalent that it should now be considered as a disease in its own right, as well as causing increased susceptibility to diabetes, cardiovascular disease and other disorders. Undernutrition, although most obvious in the developing world, also occurs in western society among vulnerable groups, particularly the elderly. Both under- and overnutrition are closely linked to illness and disease processes, affecting both the response to medical treatments and eventual recovery.

This report is a wake-up call to the medical profession to take clinical nutrition seriously. Its recommendations for nutritional assessment of all patients, for preventive measures when patients are seen to be at risk of becoming too thin or too fat, and its emphasis on the importance of well organised treatment when under- or overnutrition are sufficient to affect clinical outcome, are relevant to the practice of every clinician. The report covers both community and hospital care, and rightly emphasises the importance of teamwork across all the relevant health disciplines.

The report's recommendations are set in the context of clinical governance as a guide for the essential contribution of policy makers. They also highlight deficiencies in medical education and continued professional training which need the attention of medical schools and those responsible for postgraduate training, including this Royal College. The College will take seriously its responsibility to ensure the recommendations of this report are addressed – to do otherwise is not in the best interest of patients or society as a whole.

July 2002

Professor Sir George Alberti
President,
Royal College of Physicians

Executive summary

Introduction

Increased awareness of the hazards of under- and overnutrition has brought clinical nutrition to the fore during the last decade, as shown by the large number of publications produced on the subject. Despite this interest, clinical nutrition is often not integrated into routine clinical practice and training. This report therefore has two aims:

- To influence clinical practice, particularly by doctors, and thereby improve patient care
- To encourage all organisations responsible for health care professionals to increase their involvement in nutritional issues, through education, training and provision of patient care.

Although the report focuses on the responsibility of doctors for the nutritional care of patients, it should be read in the context of a multidisciplinary approach within both community and hospital settings. The report highlights the impact of undernutrition and overnutrition on disease processes, the influence of illness on nutrition, and the potential for nutritional intervention to contribute to disease management and prevention. The report makes recommendations for clinical governance in order to address potential shortcomings in patient care and provide methods for improving the nutritional knowledge and skills of doctors.

The membership of the working party for the report included expert representatives from health professions involved in clinical nutrition (see Appendix 1).

Recommendations

1 All doctors should be aware of nutritional problems and how to manage them. Every doctor should recognise that proper nutritional care is fundamental to good clinical practice.

2 A doctor should be responsible for ensuring that adequate information concerning nutritional status is documented in a patient's clinical record, and that appropriate action has been taken to deal with any nutritional problem.

3 Nutritional screening of all patients should be an integral part of clinical practice. Screening is a rapid process that will identify

patients who are overnourished or undernourished. If an abnormality is detected, further assessment and a specific management policy should follow.

4   Doctors should encourage patients and their families to avoid becoming overweight and assist those who are overweight to lose weight. Similarly doctors should play a key role in the detection and management of undernutrition.

5   Primary care, hospitals, nursing and residential homes should develop explicit protocols and standards to cover the whole process of nutritional management.

6   Hospitals should have a multidisciplinary nutrition steering group to establish policies for nutritional care. Doctors should be actively involved in this development. In addition, doctors should play an active role in a multidisciplinary support team for the care of patients with complicated undernutrition and patients requiring long-term tube feeds or parenteral nutrition.

7   Those responsible for clinical governance should identify nutrition as an important aspect of clinical practice that involves caterers and many health care disciplines. The inadequate provision of nutritional care has both medico-legal and ethical implications.

8   The process and outcomes of nutritional care should be part of regular clinical audit.

9   Medical undergraduate and continuing professional training programmes for doctors should include relevant aspects of clinical nutrition, along with consideration of the inter-relationships between under- and overnutrition, and illness and health. Undergraduate and postgraduate examinations should include both written and practical evaluations of nutritional knowledge.

10 The Royal College of Physicians should build on its capacity to educate, contribute to public debate and influence national policy by:

■   recognising and bringing together those with a special interest in nutrition

■   encouraging the development of knowledge about nutrition within the medical profession

■   acknowledging the importance of multiprofessional involvement for effective nutritional care

■   encouraging doctors to champion nutrition and nutritional care within NHS trusts.

Glossary

Arm muscle area
An indication of muscle bulk in the upper arm derived from measurement of the circumference of the upper arm and the thickness of subcutaneous fat measured as a skin fold.

Body Mass Index (BMI)
An index of nutritional state that takes account of both body weight and height. It is expressed as body weight (kg) divided by the square of height (m^2).

Clinical nutrition
The diagnosis and management of nutritional factors contributing to human illness.

Dysphagia
Difficulty in swallowing due to poor co-ordination or weakness of the muscles involved in the swallowing reflex, or an obstruction to the passage of food through the pharynx or gullet.

Enteral nutrition
Any technique that involves the introduction of nutrients directly into the stomach or upper small intestine through a tube.

Human nutrition
Nutritional factors in human physiology and well being.

Intestinal failure
An inability of the small intestine to absorb sufficient nutrients to maintain health.

Malabsorption
An inability of the small intestine to absorb nutrients normally.

Malnutrition
A state of nutrition in which a deficiency, excess or imbalance of energy, protein or other nutrients, including minerals and vitamins, causes measurable adverse effects on body function and clinical outcome.

Medicinal supplement

In this report, the term refers to a balanced liquid or semi-solid feed prepared commercially, available in sterile portions, and authorised for prescription in the NHS by the Advisory Committee on Borderline Substances for use on medical grounds in specified disorders including malabsorption, dysphagia and disease-related malnutrition. Liquid preparations can be used as a complete or partial source of nutrition given orally or through an enteral tube.

Nasogastric tube feed

A fine tube is introduced through the nose and pharynx so that its tip lies in the stomach. Liquid nutrients are infused through the tube either continuously using a pump or intermittently (bolus feed).

Obesity

An excess of body fat associated with a Body Mass Index greater than 30.

Overnutrition

The state of nutrition in which there is an excess of energy stores, represented by body fatness, causing measurable adverse effects on body function and clinical outcome.

Parenteral nutrition

The infusion of nutrients through a needle or cannula directly into a vein, so by-passing the gut. For short-term use, a peripheral vein can be used. For long-term treatment, the tip of the cannula needs to be situated in a large vein near the heart. The main dangers of the technique are blood-borne infection (septicaemia), clotting of blood around the tip of the cannula or metabolic complications.

Percutaneous gastrostomy

A tube is introduced through the abdominal wall so that its tip lies in the stomach, or less commonly, in the upper small intestine. The procedure is carried out under sedation using endoscopic or radiological control. The percutaneous endoscopic gastrostomy (PEG) technique involves passage of an endoscope through the mouth so that the entry site of the tube through the stomach wall can be visualised and its passage facilitated by pulling on a thread brought out through the mouth.

'Protein–energy' malnutrition

This term is frequently used in the literature since these nutrients tend to be taken together, though it is recognised that this nutritional state refers mainly to a deficiency of energy.

Triceps skin fold

A measurement of the thickness of subcutaneous fat derived from measuring the thickness of a skin fold in a standard position using calipers that exert a constant pressure.

Undernutrition

The state of nutrition in which there is a deficiency of energy, protein and other nutrients, including minerals and vitamins, causing measurable adverse effects on body function and clinical outcome.

PART ONE

Overview

1 | The relevance of nutrition to clinical practice

SUMMARY

▪ Undernutrition, overnutrition and the nutritional balance of a patient are important clinical problems commonly overlooked or ignored by doctors.

▪ Both under- and overnutrition are associated with important public health problems and significant clinical consequences at all ages.

▪ Body weight is an indicator of chronic energy balance; rapid loss of body tissue may result in important adverse physiological and psychological consequences.

▪ Correction of under- and overnutrition yields measurable clinical benefits.

▪ All doctors, whether in training or clinical practice, must recognise and manage disorders of nutrition and their consequences.

1.1 Background

Doctors' knowledge of nutrition and its clinical relevance remains poor. Surveys repeatedly confirm evidence of undernutrition in significant numbers of hospital patients, many of whom are already nutritionally depleted on admission and become more so during their hospital stay.[1] By contrast, outcome is improved in undernourished patients who are referred for nutritional treatment. Obesity is also associated with poor outcome but most physicians receive little or no training in managing obese patients – a situation that urgently needs to be addressed, given the dramatic increase in the prevalence of obesity in the UK during the past two decades.

Teaching of nutrition to undergraduates in medical school has suffered from lack of co-ordination between the different disciplines involved and is therefore not recognised as a clinical entity.[2] This has arisen because many clinical teachers themselves have had little or no training in the subject and so tend not to teach it. As a result, many doctors neglect clinical nutrition through lack of awareness of the potential benefits of nutritional care in the prevention and treatment of disease.

Poor provision of food in hospitals and evidence of undernutrition in hospital patients are common. An important step towards identifying the reasons for this came in 1992 with the publication of the King's Fund Centre's report, *A positive approach to nutrition as treatment*,[3] which showed that illness is frequently associated with undernutrition and that appropriate nutritional support confers clinical benefit. It also documented the deficiencies in care that contribute to disease-related undernutrition and how these could be remedied. The potential savings for the NHS from appropriate use of nutritional support are substantial. A recent review on behalf of the Nuffield Trust[4] succinctly summarises recommendations from the many reports on hospital nutrition published during the last decade.

A report from the National Audit Office, *Tackling obesity in England*,[5] highlights the increasing prevalence of overweight and obesity. It acknowledges that overnutrition is not an easy problem to tackle, even though modest weight loss confers significant benefits. The report suggests that part of the solution will be the *prevention* of the condition, and also recommends that health care professionals within the NHS should identify patients who are at risk from being overweight or obese, and the implementation of guidelines for the care of such patients. The problem of an escalating prevalence of obesity is not confined to the UK; a recent review published by the World Health Organisation (WHO) confirms the increasing prevalence of obesity in both the developed and developing world.[6]

This report highlights the importance of nutrition as part of good clinical practice. It identifies important areas for consideration in the training of doctors and their continuing professional education, to ensure that the nutritional care of patients is always addressed as part of their overall management.

The report is not intended to review extensively or provide detailed guidance for the nutritional management of patients. Although the report emanates from the Royal College of Physicians, its recommendations on medical training are relevant to all doctors and to the totality of patient care: the symptoms and signs of nutritional imbalance are frequently multiple and non-specific, cross all medical disciplines and are often entirely attributable to the underlying disease. The non-specific nature of nutritional imbalance partly accounts for the failure of doctors to recognise and treat under- and overnutrition. Whilst the report is directed to the care of adult patients, the principles addressed are just as relevant to infants and children with under- or overnutrition.

1.2 What is malnutrition?

Malnutrition may be defined as a state of nutrition in which a deficiency, excess or imbalance of energy, protein or other nutrients, including minerals and vitamins, causes measurable adverse effects on body function and clinical outcome. Malnutrition may affect a wide range of body functions including physical activity, reproductive ability, cognitive ability and the response to disease and infection.[7] All of these factors impact on the overall quality of a person's life. Vitamin deficiencies may occur in particular conditions, such as alcoholism, over-restrictive diets, and in older people who are socially isolated.

The adverse effects of malnutrition respond to nutritional intervention, although some effects of long-term malnutrition may be irreversible.

For definitions of other general terms used in the report, see Box 1.1. See also Glossary, p. xi.

Box 1.1   Definitions

Human nutrition: Nutritional factors in human physiology and well-being.

Clinical nutrition: The diagnosis and management of nutritional factors contributing to human illness.

Malnutrition: A state of nutrition in which a deficiency, excess or imbalance of energy, protein or other nutrients, including minerals and vitamins, causes measurable adverse effects on body function and clinical outcome.

Undernutrition: The state of nutrition in which there is a deficiency of energy, protein and other nutrients, including minerals and vitamins, causing measurable adverse effects on body function and clinical outcome.

'Protein–energy' malnutrition: This term is frequently used in the literature since these nutrients tend to be taken together, though it is recognised that this nutritional state mainly refers to a deficiency of energy.

Overnutrition: The state of nutrition in which there is an excess of energy stores, represented by body fatness, causing measurable adverse effects on body function and clinical outcome.

Obesity: An excess of body fat associated with a Body Mass Index greater than 30.

1.3 Body weight as a broad indicator of chronic energy imbalance

In clinical practice, body weight as a measure of health is expressed by using a formula that combines weight and height. The underlying assumption is that most variation in a person's body weight at the same height is due to fat mass.[6,7] The formula most frequently used is Body Mass Index (BMI), which is weight in kilograms divided by the square of the height in metres. BMI is strongly correlated with densitometry measurements of percentage fat mass, adjusted for height in middle-aged adults. The main limitation of BMI is that it does not distinguish fat mass from lean mass; it may additionally be misleading if there is oedema or a neurological cause of muscle wasting.

A graded classification for BMI is valuable in clinical practice for a number of reasons:

▪ It provides a meaningful comparison of weight status within and between patients.

▪ It identifies individuals and groups of patients at increased risk of morbidity and mortality.

▪ It identifies individual patients who should be prioritised for nutritional intervention.

Table 1.1 provides a categorisation of BMI to assess whether patients are at risk from malnutrition.

Table 1.1 Classification of BMI to assess patients at risk from malnutrition

Classification	BMI category (kg/m^2)	Significance
Underweight	<18.5	Chronic protein–energy undernutrition probable
Lower end of normal range – borderline underweight	18.5 – <20	Chronic protein–energy undernutrition possible
Normal range	20 – <25	Chronic protein–energy undernutrition unlikely
Overweight – pre-obese	25 – <30	Increased risk of co-morbidities related to chronic energy overnutrition
Obese class 1	30 – <35	Moderate risk of co-morbidities
Obese class 2	35 – <40	Severe risk of co-morbidities
Obese class 3	40 or greater	Very severe risk of co-morbidities

Ideally, body weight and height should be measured using calibrated weighing scales and an accurate stadiometer. BMI may not correspond to the same degree of fatness and thinness across different populations.

Note that these BMI values are age-independent and the same for both men and women. BMI increases with age and, at a given BMI, women have more body fat than men. Importantly, the categorisation of risk can be overridden by clinical judgement – for example, some perfectly healthy adults are constitutionally thin and have a BMI of 18.5–20. The estimation of BMI is relevant only to chronic protein–energy status and does not take account of those individuals who have become undernourished and have lost body function as a result of considerable, unintentional, recent weight loss.

Acute nutritional deficiency independent of BMI

Clinicians should also be aware that patients may suffer from acute energy deficiency with adverse functional consequences even though the BMI may remain within or above the normal range. An example is seen in surgical practice during the peri-operative period, when acute nutritional deficiency can cause muscle weakness with reduced ability to cough effectively.[8]

1.4 The clinical relevance of nutritional care

The clinical relevance of the nutritional care of patients is summarised in Box 1.2. There are few aspects of medicine in which nutritional knowledge is not important or useful.

1.5 Prevalence of under- and overnutrition in the UK

Undernutrition

In national dietary surveys, adults with a BMI <20 account for approximately 5% of the UK population.[7] The WHO has proposed a BMI of 18.5 to signify underweight, which, if applied to the UK population, means that about 2% of the adult population has a high likelihood of being undernourished.[7,18] Undernutrition can manifest itself in various ways and develop acutely or insidiously in patients with a wide variety of inflammatory and non-inflammatory problems. It can affect the function of every system of the body, producing adverse effects on physical and psychosocial well-being.

A study of the nutritional status of hospital patients by McWhirter and Pennington[1] showed that 200 of 500 (40%) consecutive admissions to an acute teaching hospital were at least mildly undernourished. Those patients who were in hospital for more than one week were reassessed on discharge. Of these, 64% had lost weight, including 75% of the 55 patients classified as undernourished on admission. In contrast, weight gain was observed in 20% of patients, but only 12.5% of those were originally classified as undernourished. The correspondence that followed the publication of this paper indicated similar findings from surveys in other UK hospitals, although the frequency of undernutrition ranged from 13% to 40% depending on the definition applied.[19]

Overnutrition

Despite the clinical importance of undernutrition, overweight and obesity are now the major nutritional disorders affecting the developed

> ## Box 1.2   The clinical relevance of nutritional care
>
> **Malnutrition in the developing world** – this is an enormous problem of world health, but outside the scope of this report.
>
> **Heart disease, cancer, obesity, diabetes and bone disease** – these increasingly prevalent problems, characteristic of the developed world and urban centres in the developing world, have a major nutritional component.
>
> **Undernourished patients in Britain** – up to 40% of hospital admissions and 10% of patients in primary care suffer undernutrition,[1,9] but despite the availability of effective treatment malnutrition goes largely unrecognised and untreated, leading to worse outcome from disease, prolonging convalescence and escalating health care costs. In the UK, 12.4% of the population living in the community aged 65 years or older are at medium or high risk of undernutrition, rising to 20.5% of those of comparable age living in residential accommodation.
>
> **Nutrition in pregnancy and early life** – both low and high maternal BMI is related to low or high birth weight and an increased chance of neonatal morbidity and mortality. Foetal, perinatal and childhood nutrition affects not only mental and physical development, but also may influence health in later life.[10,11,12]
>
> **Later life** – nutrition influences the ageing process, bone disease and general health in old age.[13]
>
> **Immune function** – there is growing evidence that the development and function of the immune system may be influenced by nutritional factors both early and late in life.[14]
>
> **Pharmacology** – the absorption and action of drugs are influenced by nutrition. Some drugs cause an increase in weight through their effect on appetite (eg phenothiazines and corticosteroids). In turn, drugs may affect nutritional status by causing nausea, influencing nutrient absorption, or altering vitamin metabolism, particularly in the elderly; examples include paracetamol, anticonvulsant medication and digoxin.[15]
>
> **Surgery** – outcomes of surgery and rehabilitation are influenced by diet and nutritional state.[16,17]
>
> **Prevention and treatment** – most of the above problems are amenable to nutritional treatment or prevention, which in turn depend on better knowledge and understanding on the part of doctors and nurses.[3,4,7,9]

world and are also emerging as significant problems in developing nations. The WHO recognised the problem of overnutrition for the first time in 1997 when it concluded: 'The epidemic projections for the next decade are so serious that public health action is urgently required'.[6] Obesity, defined as a BMI >30, is now of such importance that it deserves to be considered as a disease in its own right and therefore managed like any other chronic disease, with a programme of detection and continued support and follow-up.

The most comprehensive information on prevalence of overweight and obesity in Europe comes from the data collected between 1983 and 1986 for the MONICA study.[20] On average, 15% of men and 22% of women were obese, with overweight being much more common in women than men. More than half the adults between 35 and 65 years of age in Europe were either overweight or obese. In England and Wales, the most recent health survey has confirmed an increase in the prevalence of obesity in adults from 6% in men and 8% in women in 1980 to 17% of men and 21% of women in 1998.[21] The changes in adult prevalence of overweight and obesity are reflected by an even more striking change in childhood and adolescence in both industrialised and developing countries. The early onset of obesity increases the likelihood of obesity in later life, as well as the prevalence of obesity-related disorders (see section 1.8). Childhood factors implicated in the development of adult obesity therefore have far-reaching implications for costs to the health service and the economy.[22]

1.6 Complications of undernutrition

Undernutrition adversely affects a wide range of physical functions as a consequence of both acute and chronic protein–energy deprivation.[3,7,8] These changes include:

- impaired immune responses, predisposing to infection
- reduced muscle strength and increased fatiguability, contributing to inactivity, inability to work effectively and poor self-care. Abnormal muscle function may predispose to falls
- reduced respiratory muscle strength and fatigue leading to poor cough pressure, predisposing to and delaying recovery from chest infection
- inactivity, especially in bed-bound patients, predisposing to sores and thromboembolism
- impaired thermoregulation leading to hypothermia, especially in the elderly
- impaired wound healing and prolonged recovery from illness, increased length of hospital stay and delayed return to work.

Undernutrition, even when not accompanied by disease, tends to cause apathy, depression, self neglect, hypochondriasis, loss of libido and deterioration in social interactions.

Individuals are affected by undernutrition in different ways, depending on their age, initial body weight and the degree of pre-existing impairment of body function caused by specific disease. The association between malnutrition and poor clinical outcome is not confined to surgical patients. In medical patients, malnutrition is a precursor of complications during hospital stay, and the risk of elderly patients developing complications is correlated with nutritional status before admission. Patients with acute illness, including stroke, cardiac and respiratory failure, are more likely to die if they are malnourished.

1.7 Benefits of correcting undernutrition

A number of studies show a relationship between nutritional status and clinical outcomes. For example, two randomised control trials of nutritional support demonstrated improved outcomes in patients undergoing orthopaedic surgery, and a reduction in major complications and mortality.[26,27] Those patients given oral supplements had fewer complications – such as pressure sores, wound infections with anaemia – and lower mortality than those who received no supplements.

Patients with malnutrition, in particular those patients who are malnourished on admission, stay in hospital longer, although it can be difficult to dissociate this from the severity of illness.[28–31] However, systematic reviews have not shown consistent evidence for substantial clinical benefit from measures to improve nutrition due to the inclusion of poorly designed studies in which there was:

▪ failure to stratify patients by nutritional status on entry to or during the study, resulting in uncertainties as to whether the nutritional intervention was efficacious

▪ failure to take account of confounding factors, especially co-morbidity and non-compliance, resulting in uncertainties as to whether the nutritional intervention was effective.

Such issues need to be addressed in future studies.

Box 1.3 outlines the clinical benefits that may follow the provision of nutritional support.

1.8 Complications of overnutrition

There is a close relationship between BMI and the incidence of several chronic conditions caused by excess fat: type II diabetes, hypertension, coronary heart disease and cholelithiasis.[23] This relationship is approximately linear for a range of BMI indexes less than 30: American women with a BMI of 26 have a two-fold greater risk of coronary heart disease compared to women with a BMI of less than 21. They have an eight-fold greater risk of developing type II diabetes.[24] The equivalent figures for American men are a 1.5-fold increase and a four-fold increase respectively. The risk of hypertension is doubled in both men and women with a BMI of 26. All risks are greatly increased for those

> **Box 1.3 Provision of nutritional support for undernourished patients improves clinical outcome**[9,28,32,33, 33a]
>
> ▪ Nutritional support maintains or improves nutritional status and other intermediate biomarkers
>
> ▪ A number of studies have demonstrated clinical benefits of nutritional supplementation in terms of rate of complications, length of stay, and/or mortality ·
>
> ▪ Studies that have examined the clinical benefits of short-term nutritional support in the community and the available evidence suggest improved functional status and quality of life
>
> ▪ In most cases, enteral and parenteral nutrition are effective in different circumstances. It is generally accepted that enteral nutrition should be used whenever possible – both therapies can be life-saving in patients who cannot eat normal foods over a long period.

subjects with a BMI of more than 29, regardless of gender.[25] A list of conditions causally related to overweight and obesity is given in Box 1.4.

1.9 Benefits of correcting overnutrition

An important recognition of recent years in the management of obesity has been the impact of a 5–10% weight loss in terms of improving an individual's risk profile. This is a goal that for some is both achievable and sustainable, and can have a major impact in reducing the mortality and morbidity associated with obesity. Box 1.5 lists the potential medical benefits for patients who achieve modest weight loss.

The benefits of physical activity should also be considered, and where possible exercise should be included as part of weight management. Physical activity represents approximately 15–20% of the total daily energy expenditure (see Fig 1). Any increase in physical activity

> **Box 1.4 Chronic conditions that are causally related to overweight and obesity**
>
> ▪ Metabolic disorders (type II diabetes mellitus and dyslipidaemias)
>
> ▪ Cardiovascular disease and hypertension
>
> ▪ Respiratory problems (most notably obstructive sleep apnoea)
>
> ▪ Certain cancers
>
> ▪ Musculoskeletal problems (in particular osteoarthritis)
>
> ▪ Gastrointestinal disorders (including gall stones and oesophageal reflux)
>
> ▪ Reproductive disorders (including infertility)
>
> ▪ Psychological disorders

Box 1.5 Health benefits achievable from 5–10% weight loss in an obese person[34-40]

▌ Symptoms of angina reduced by 91%

▌ 33% increase in exercise tolerance

▌ Fall of 30–50% in fasting plasma glucose

▌ Fall of 10 mmHg systolic and diastolic pressures

▌ Fall by 15% in LDL; fall by 30% in triglyceride; increase by 8% in HDL cholesterol

▌ Marked improvement in both quality and quantity of sleep with reduced snoring

▌ Marked improvement in mobility and reduction in pain

▌ Increased regularity of menstrual cycle and improved fertility

LDL = low density lipoprotein; HDL = high density lipoprotein.

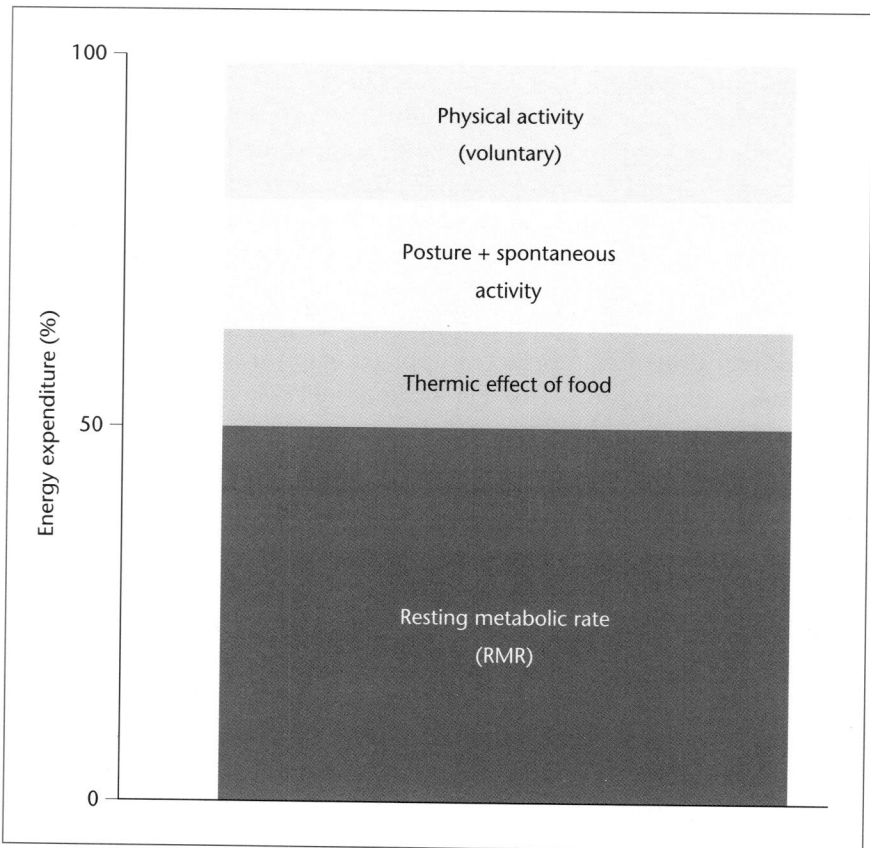

Figure 1 The components of daily energy expenditure expressed as percentages.

will therefore contribute to an increase in expenditure and may assist with weight loss. Although the amount of weight loss achieved by physical activity is modest (0.5 to 1 kg per month), the associated physiological benefits to an individual are substantial. Physical activity should always be considered as a component of a weight loss programme; it may be particularly helpful for maintaining weight loss.

1.10 Under- and overnutrition in older people

Nutritional problems are common in older people. Table 1.2 shows percentages of those aged 65 years and over who were found to be overweight (BMI >25) or who showed evidence of undernutrition (BMI <20), in the most recently published UK National Diet and Nutrition Survey (NDNS).[41] This table illustrates the magnitude of the problem in a growing elderly population and reflects the greater frailty of individuals living in care. It is essential to consider nutritional well-being as part of the care of the older patient.

Individuals who have evidence of acute or chronic weight loss are also at risk of vitamin and trace element deficiencies. Individuals in long-term care are at particular risk, especially of vitamin D, iron, folate and vitamin C deficiency.[41]

Table 1.2 Percentage of people 65 years and over in the UK who are either underweight or overweight[41]

Status	Underweight: BMI <20		Overweight: BMI >25	
	Men (%)	Women (%)	Men (%)	Women (%)
Independent in community	3	6	63	67
Living in care	16	15	46	47

1.11 Factors influencing the increase in malnutrition in hospital and in the community

The Nuffield Trust report, *Managing nutrition in hospital*,[4] confirmed an urgent need to tackle malnutrition at all levels of the NHS; it further confirmed widespread support for the proposal that food provision should be considered as part of clinical care, with management and accountability through the clinical line. The report also highlighted the importance of clearly defining roles and responsibilities regarding nutritional care at ward level, of quality assurance and co-ordination at senior management level within each trust.

There are important medico-legal and ethical implications implicit within the provision of adequate nutritional care. Some of the recommendations have been addressed within the NHS Plan,[42] but scant attention has been given to the specific training needs of doctors and allied health professions. It is disappointing that doctors do not regard nutrition as important, particularly when correction of nutritional imbalance results in appreciable benefit to the patient (see Box 1.2). Malnutrition will continue in many patients, both in hospital and the community, until the following issues have been addressed:

- lack of training and knowledge
- lack of interest
- the scarcity of specialists with necessary skills and knowledge
- inadequate hospital management policies for nutrition and nutritional care and for the provision of hospital food
- the need for better organisation of nutritional services within trusts.

This report aims to address these issues and to establish nutrition as an essential part of patient care.

References

1 McWhirter JP, Pennington CR. Incidence and recognition of malnutrition in hospital. *BMJ* 1994; **308**: 945–8.

2 Jackson AA. Human nutrition in medical practice: the training of doctors. *Proceedings of the Nutrition Society* 2001; **61**: 257–63.

3 Lennard-Jones JE (ed). *A positive approach to nutrition as treatment: report of a working party on the role of enteral and parenteral feeding in hospital and home.* London: King's Fund Centre, 1992.

4 Maryon Davis A, Bristow A. *Managing nutrition in hospital: a recipe for quality.* London: The Nuffield Trust, 1999.

5 National Audit Office. *Tackling obesity in England: report by the Comptroller and Auditor General.* London: The Stationery Office, 2001.

6 World Health Organisation. *Obesity: preventing and managing the global epidemic. Report of a WHO consultation on obesity.* Geneva: World Health Organisation, 1998.

7 Elia M (ed). *Guidelines for the detection and management of malnutrition.* Redditch: Malnutrition Advisory Group, The British Association for Parenteral and Enteral Nutrition, 2000.

8 Windsor JA, Hill GL. Weight loss with physiologic impairment. *Ann Surg* 1988; **207**: 290–96.

9 Green CJ. Existence, causes and consequences of disease-related malnutrition in the hospital and the community, and clinical and financial benefits of nutritional intervention. *Eur J Clin Nutr* 1999; **18**(suppl.2): 3–28.

10 Allen LH, Lun'aho MS, Shaheen M *et al.* Maternal body mass index and pregnancy outcome in the Nutrition Collaborative Support Program. *Eur J Clin Nutr* 1994; **48**(suppl.3): S68–S77.

11 Barker DJP. Foetal origins of coronary heart disease. *BMJ* 1995; **311**: 171–4.

12 Sebire NJ, Jolly M, Harris JP *et al.* Maternal obesity and pregnancy outcome: a

study of 287,213 pregnancies in London. *Int J Obes Relat Metab Disord* 2001; **25**: 1175–82.

13 Sullivan DH, Sun S, Wallis RC. Protein-energy undernutrition among elderly hospitalised patients. *J Am Med Assoc* 1999; **281**: 2013–19.

14 Chandra RK, Kumari S. Effects of nutrition on the immune system. *Nutrition* 1994; **10**: 207–210.

15 Thomas JA. Drug-nutrient interactions. *Nutr Rev* 1995; **53**: 271–81.

16 Warnold I, Lundholm K. Clinical significance of preoperative nutritional status in 215 noncancer patients. *Ann Surg* 1984; **201**: 299–305.

17 Windsor JA, Knight GS, Hill GL. Wound healing response in surgical patients: recent food intake is more important than nutritional status. *Br J Surg* 1988; **75**: 135–7.

18 Elia M, Lunn PG. Biological markers of protein energy malnutrition. *Eur J Clin Nutr* 1997; **16**(suppl.1): 11–17.

19 Kelly IE, Tessier S, Cahill A, *et al.* Still hungry in hospital: identifying malnutrition in acute hospital admissions. *QJM* 2000; **93**: 93–8.

20 World Health Organisation. MONICA Project: geographical variation in the major risk factors of coronary heart disease in men and women aged 35–64 years. *World Health Stat Q* 1988; **41**: 115–40.

21 Joint Health Surveys Unit (on behalf of the Department of Health). *Health Survey for England: cardiovascular disease 1998*. London: The Stationery Office, 1999.

22 Parsons TJ, Power C, Logan S, Summerbell CD. Childhood predictors of adult obesity: a systematic review. *Int J Obes* 1999; **23**(Suppl 8): S1–S107.

23 Kopelman PG. Obesity as a medical problem. *Nature* 2000; **404**: 635–43.

24 Hubert HB. The importance of obesity in the development of coronary risk factors and disease: the epidemiological evidence. *Ann Rev Public Health* 1986; **7**: 493–502.

25 Willett WC, Dietz WH, Colditz GA. Guidelines for healthy weight. *N Eng J Med* 1999; **341**: 427–33.

26 Bastow MD, Rawlings J, Allison SP. Benefits of supplementary tube feeding after fractured neck of femur. A randomised control trial. *BMJ* 1983; **287**: 1589–92.

27 Delmi M, Rapin CH, Bengoa JM *et al.* Dietary supplementation in elderly patients with fractured neck of the femur. *Lancet* 1990; **335**: 1013–16.

28 Forman H. Relationship of malnutrition and length of stay in hospital. *J Am Diet Assoc* 1996; **96**(Suppl): 29.

29 Treber LA, Harris MA. Effect of early nutrition intervention on patient length of stay. *J Am Diet Ass* 1996; **96**(Suppl): 29.

30 Tucker HN, Miguel SG. Cost containment through nutrition intervention. *Nutr Rev* 1996; **54**: 111–21.

31 Klein S, Kinney J, Jeejeebhoy K *et al.* Nutrition support in clinical practice: review of published data and recommendations for future research directions. *J Parenteral Enteral Nutrition* 1997; **21**: 133–56.

32 Stratton RJ, Elia M. A critical systematic analysis of the use of oral nutritional supplements in the community. *Eur J Clin Nutr* 1999; **18**(Suppl 2): 29–84.

33 Christie PM, Hill GL. Effect of intravenous nutrition on nutrition and functions in acute attacks of inflammatory bowel disease. *Gastroenterology* 1990; **99**: 730–36.

33a Jamieson CP, Norton B, Day T, Lakeman M, Powell-Tuck J. The quantitative effect of nutrition support on quantity of life in outpatients. *Clin Nutr* 1997; **16**: 25–8.

34 Williamson DF, Pamuk E, Thun M *et al.* Prospective study of intentional weight loss and mortality in never smoking, overweight, US white women aged 40-64 years. *Am J Epidemiol* 1995; **141**: 1128–34.

35 Van Gaal LF, Wauters MA, De Leeuw IH. The beneficial effects of modest weight loss on cardiovascular risk factors. *Int J Obes* 1997; **21**: 55–9.

36 Reisen E, Abel R, Modan M *et al.* The effect of weight loss without salt restriction on the reduction in blood pressure in overweight hypertensive patients. *N Engl J Med* 1978; **298**: 1–6.

37 Lean MEJ, Hankey CR . Benefits and risks of weight loss. In: Kopelman PG, Stock MJ (eds) *Clinical obesity.* Oxford: Blackwell Science, 1998: 564–96.

38 Smith PL, Gold AR, Myers DA *et al.* Weight loss in mildly to moderately obese patients with obstructive sleep apnoea. *Ann Intern Med* 1985; **103**: 850–55.

39 McGoey BV, Deital M, Saplys RJ, Kliman ME. Effect of weight loss on musculoskeletal pain in the morbidly obese. *J Bone Joint Surg Br* 1990; **72**: 322–23.

40 Kiddy DS, Hamilton-Fairley D, Bush A *et al.* Improvement in endocrine and ovarian function during dietary restriction of obese women with polycystic ovary syndrome. *Clin Endocrinol* 1992; **36**: 105–11.

41 Finch S, Doyle W, Lowe C *et al. National Diet and Nutrition Survey: people aged 65 years and over. Volume 1: report of the diet and nutrition survey.* London: The Stationery Office, 1998.

42 Department of Health. *The NHS Plan: a plan for investment, a plan for reform.* London: Stationery Office, 2000.

2 | What all doctors need to know

SUMMARY

- Doctors should understand the clinical importance of a balanced diet, of patients being under- or overweight or of being deprived of nutrients for even a period of days, and of specific nutritional deficiencies.
- Doctors need to recognise nutritional deficiency or excess and quantify them when possible.
- Nutritional care depends on team work between health care workers in different disciplines, the scope and contribution of whose work should be recognised.
- Communication within each health care team and between teams in the community and in hospital is essential.
- Ethical considerations regarding nutritional care are important for all involved, but especially for doctors who are called upon to make decisions about nutritional treatment of patients unable to take such decisions for themselves.

2.1 Diet: excess and deficiency

A balanced diet

The Government regularly issues dietary advice and seeks to educate the population in healthy eating habits, encouraging an increase in fruit, vegetable and cereal consumption, and a decrease in fat intake. The most sustained publicity campaign in recent years was the Health of the Nation Task Force which has now completed its programme of recommendations and publications (see Appendix 2). It is important that doctors are familiar with the evidence for an alteration in the national dietary habits so that they can answer patients' enquiries on nutrition and healthy eating.

Deficient energy intake

Two types of energy depletion can be recognised – chronic protein–energy deficiency, shown by a low BMI, and acute undernutrition evidenced by recent unintended weight loss. The former is well recognised but there is increasing evidence that acute deprivation of food for even hours or days has adverse functional consequences.[1]

Healthy people who starve (such as hunger strikers) for 6–8 weeks lose approximately one-third of their body weight before death occurs, as illustrated in Fig 2. A person who has undergone trauma, or suffers from any illness that induces a catabolic response, loses weight more rapidly, so that 10% weight loss can occur in 15 days and 20% in 26 days,[2] and death supervenes earlier. The weight loss is clinically more serious if the person is already undernourished because there is less tissue reserve to draw upon. Experimentally, healthy people who take two-thirds or less of their usual energy intake lose weight progressively so that after six months it has fallen by almost a quarter.[2] This state of undernutrition is accompanied by muscle weakness, depression and apathy as described in Chapter 1, section 1.6. As during total starvation, these changes develop more rapidly if a person's metabolism is catabolic due to trauma or illness.[2]

These facts are clinically important in all types of medicine and, as shown in Fig 2, therapeutic decisions about nutritional support are needed when a patient has lost 5–10% of normal body weight and further loss is likely to occur.

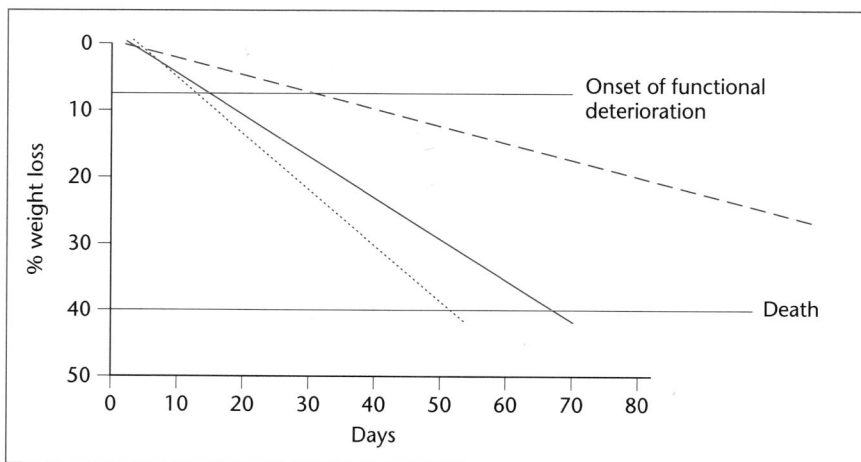

Figure 2 The figure shows the rate of weight loss experienced by otherwise healthy subjects undergoing semi-starvation (- - - - -), otherwise healthy subjects undergoing complete starvation (————), and catabolic patients with severe illness or trauma undergoing semi-starvation (··············). Ill patients lose weight when nutritionally depleted at a faster rate than otherwise healthy subjects. Functional deterioration and tissue loss become clinically significant when 5–10% of body weight is lost. Death from starvation occurs when approximately 40% of body weight is lost. Modified from Ref 2.

Excess energy intake

Excess energy intake leads to accumulation of body fat with the potential clinical consequences described in Chapter 1, section 1.8.

Specific deficiencies

The importance of folic acid supplements during pregnancy in reducing foetal spinal defects is now well recognised. Low blood levels of vitamin D occur, particularly among the elderly, due to lack of exposure to sunlight and poor dietary intake (see section 3.7 below). Thiamine deficiency can complicate alcoholism. Deficiency of other vitamins is usually a complication of a severely restricted diet.

Adequate calcium intake is important (see section 3.7 below). There is evidence that dietary intake, blood levels and whole body levels of selenium are falling in Europe, but the significance of these observations is not clear. Selenium is a constituent of anti-oxidant enzymes, is important in thyroid hormone synthesis and in male reproductive function.[3]

2.2 Screening for nutritional 'risk'

The first essential is to recognise whether a patient is under- or overnourished. This is a quick process, easily achieved by simple observation, which will identify patients at nutritional risk, defined as those in whom:

▪ nutritional factors are likely to affect clinical outcomes such as bodily functions, sense of well-being, rate of recovery, length of hospital stay and survival; and

▪ nutritional intervention (support in undernutrition or weight loss in obesity) is likely to affect clinical outcome.

Use of screening tools to assess undernutrition

A number of screening tools are in use, or are being developed,[4] to assess undernutrition. The basic elements of the screening process should address the following questions which relate to continuity of care:

▪ *Where is the patient now?* Height, weight, BMI and severity of illness; in children, the screening tool will also involve measurement of growth rate.

▪ *Where has the patient come from?* Recent weight change.

▪ *Where is the patient going?* Effects of disease and proposed treatments on food intake in relation to likely requirements, which in turn depend on the metabolic response to disease and its effect on metabolic rate.

Each screening tool categorises patients. The addition of risk factors will give a numerical score (see Fig 3) which will indicate whether nutritional help is needed and the type of management that is appropriate, but it should not be followed slavishly. All screening data need to be interpreted intelligently in the light of clinical knowledge and experience, and care plans should be adapted to circumstances, for example in the care of a patient with dementia or comfort for a person who is dying (see section 2.7).

In acutely ill or bed-ridden patients it is not always possible to measure height and weight, so this information may sometimes be obtained by enquiry from the patient or family. In other cases, for example some older patients, surrogate measures of height (eg tibial length or demispan) and lean body mass (eg mid-arm circumference) may be useful, or the fact that a patient's clothes or jewellery have become loose may give evidence of weight loss. Sometimes a qualitative estimate only is possible, noting that the patient is obese, normal, thin or very thin. If the patient's condition later permits, measurements should be made and recorded. When oedema or dehydration are present, or resolving with treatment, the calculation of BMI should take account of these factors.

Definitions of terms used in nutritional assessment are given in Box 2.1.

The Malnutrition Advisory Group of the British Association for Parental and Enteral Nutrition[5] has produced a screening tool for adults at risk of malnutrition in the community which uses BMI and unintended recent weight loss as the main criteria for chronic and acute undernutrition respectively, but also allows for clinical observation (Fig 3). This type of screening tool is also being adapted for use in hospital.

Box 2.1   Definitions of terms used in nutritional assessment

Body Mass Index: An index of nutritional state that takes account of both body weight and height. It is expressed as body weight (kg) divided by the square of height (m²).

Arm muscle area: An indication of muscle bulk in the upper arm derived from measurement of the circumference of the upper arm and the thickness of subcutaneous fat measured as a skin fold.

Triceps skin fold: A measurement of the thickness of subcutaneous fat derived from measuring the thickness of a skin fold in a standard position using calipers that exert a constant pressure.

Nutritional status

Chronic		Acute
BMI (kg/m²) *Score*	*plus*	Wt loss in 3–6 months *Score*
>20.0 = 0		0 = <5%
18.5–20.0 = 1		1 = 5–10%
<18.5 = 2		2 = >10%

■ If weight and height are not available, recalled height or weight may be appropriate. Take care interpreting the patient's BMI or percent weight loss when there are fluid disturbances, muscle wasting, immobility, neurological conditions or pregnancy. If weight/height measurements are not possible, form a clinical opinion of risk from questions (eg loosely fitting clothes/rings, loss of appetite and whether improving or deteriorating).

■ Healthy adults with no weight loss (or <5%) in the previous 6 months are given a score of zero.

■ The combined score can be used as a guide to subsequent action:

Overall risk of undernutrition

	Low	Medium	High
Score	0	1	2 or more
Action	No action	Observe	Treat

Note: clinical judgement is important with respect to categorisation and treatment (see text).

Figure 3 A scoring system (screening tool) designed for use in the community to categorise the risk of undernutrition and indicate when corrective action is needed (see text). Adapted from Ref 5.

A numerical score of zero using this screening tool can give a false sense of security if the course of an illness is likely to cause major clinical deterioration. A few healthy young people have a BMI between 18.5 and 20. Continued weight loss due to illness may result in a patient in the intermediate group quickly becoming obviously undernourished. Also, even though a patient is in the high risk group, active nutritional supplementation may sometimes be inappropriate because death is imminent or the discomfort of treatment outweighs the benefit (see section 2.6).

2.3 Nutritional assessment

When the screening process has identified a patient as being 'at nutritional risk', then more detailed assessment should follow. Possible quantitative data include a detailed dietary assessment by a dietitian and possibly prospective measurements of food intake. Anthropometric measurements, such as muscle bulk or strength, or subcutaneous fat, have advantages and limitations. The normal range for some tests was established using healthy populations many years ago and may not be appropriate for patients, often in older age groups, today.[6,7,8]

Qualitative assessment includes psychological, socioeconomic and ethnic factors, as well as practical aspects affecting nutrient intake such as dentition, or an inability to swallow normally or to feed independently.

2.4 Team work – the contribution of different disciplines

It is the doctor's responsibility to understand and appreciate the crucial role of other disciplines, particularly nurses, dietitians, speech therapists and pharmacists, in the nutritional care of patients.

Nurses

The United Kingdom Central Council for Nursing, Midwifery and Health Visitors (UKCC) has issued a statement that nurses are responsible for ensuring that patients in hospital are adequately fed,[9] but their responsibilities go further than this. A wide-ranging resource pack entitled *Eating matters* has been published as a nursing initiative for the benefit not only of nurses but also of all professionals involved in nutritional care.[10] Nutrition screening, as already described, is an integral part of nurses' hospital admission procedure, and weight and nutritional state should be monitored at regular intervals during a patient's hospital stay to detect deterioration or response to treatment. Nurses in hospital should identify those who need assistance with nutrition, such as help with feeding or completing menus, and those who need special diets.

An important function of ward nurses is to co-ordinate the work of other health professionals, such as dietitians, speech therapists, occupational therapists and doctors, in the nutritional care of the patient. On discharge of the patient, nurses play a part in the communication process with the primary care team about any nutritional issues.

A clinical nurse specialist (CNS) in nutrition is often the only full-time member of a nutrition support team and thus is an expert in the management of artificial nutrition in both acute and community settings. A major function of a clinical nurse specialist is that of an educator of nursing colleagues, other health professionals, including doctors, and patients, about the techniques of artificial nutrition. Such nurses often have a wide remit with regard to patient nutrition, beyond that of artificial nutrition.

Whenever an ethical issue arises, for example the possible use of a tube feed or fluid infusion at the end of life, nurses expect to be involved as an integral part of the decision-making process, particularly as they have often formed the closest relationships with patients and their families.

Dietitians

Dietitians provide a service both in the community and hospital. They are usually the only members of the health care team who have received a dedicated and prolonged training in nutrition. The British Dietetic Association has published a position paper that defines the key role of dietitians in the prevention and treatment of malnutrition in hospital. It also emphasises their potential contribution in training other staff, including doctors at under- and postgraduate levels, in good nutritional care.[11] Through their own literature and professional meetings, they have up-to-date knowledge of current trends.

Dietetic staff are skilled at making quantitative estimates of what a patient eats and its relation to recommended standards. Similarly, they can assess the nutritional value of a diet or individual meals, a skill useful when arranging special meals for patients or specifying and monitoring the nutritional value of hospital meals when catering is based on a contract specifying minimum values.

In the care of patients, dietitians are particularly adept at offering advice that is realistic and practical, for example how undernourished patients can supplement their intake using normal food and how those who are overnourished can reduce their energy intake. They can teach other health professionals how to advise patients about simple dietary changes. This function is important because the number of dietitians in a district or hospital is usually small and it would be impossible for one of them to see every patient who needed dietary advice or a simple modification of diet.

Ideally, a dietitian in hospital should have responsibility for a specialty or a group of wards and be recognised as a person in the ward team who works closely with nursing and medical staff, and pharmacists, in developing agreed strategies for nutritional care. In the 1999/2000 Audit Commission survey, dietitians in 41% of acute hospital trusts reported that they were unable to see all patients referred.[12] It is therefore necessary that referrals should be restricted to those where a dietitian's skills are needed, but equally there is often a shortage of dietetic staff.

A dietitian is almost always a member of a nutrition support team, in approximately 10% of current teams acts as leader, and often takes particular responsibility for enteral tube feeds.[13]

Speech and language therapists

Speech and language therapists are skilled in the assessment of swallowing disorders. Their number in a district or hospital is small and they are not available outside normal working hours. Their skills should therefore be reserved for dealing with problem cases and for teaching other staff, usually nurses, to assess a patient's ability to swallow safely. Their role is to give skilled advice, but it is the doctor's responsibility to decide whether a patient with a possible swallowing disorder can be given semi-solid food, liquids or normal food without danger of aspiration.

Pharmacists

Pharmacists have an important role during nutritional support in advising on the compatibility of mixtures used for parenteral feeding and in preparing the solutions for infusion. They also advise on matters such as the administration of drugs usually given by mouth, when an enteral tube feed is being given.

2.5 Communication within and between health care teams

If a nutritional factor relevant to the clinical care of a patient is identified, this information should be passed on if a doctor transfers responsibility to a colleague. Doctors also need to communicate closely with colleagues in other disciplines regarding nutritional care plans.

The importance of good communication between hospital and primary care teams is especially important when continuity of nutritional care is needed.

2.6 Ethical considerations

Patient consent

Tube feeding is regarded in law as a medical treatment, not as part of basic care, and it requires the consent of a competent patient. If, after explanation of its purpose and any anticipated discomfort or possible complication, an adult refuses the treatment proposed, this decision is binding on the carers. If the patient does not accept what appears to be in his/her best interest, this is not a reason for regarding the patient as incompetent.[14,15] In such circumstances, a senior doctor needs to be among those who discuss the matter with the patient without putting pressure upon him/her. The outcome of the discussion should be written in the medical record.

A particularly difficult matter relating to patient consent concerns patients with such severe anorexia nervosa that their life is in danger. Under the provisions of the Mental Health Act 1983, such patients, subject to the proper procedures,[16] can be admitted against their will for treatment of their mental condition. To date, courts have decided that tube feeding constitutes an aspect of such treatment when medically advisable, but legal opinion should be sought if there is doubt in a particular case.*

Comfort at the end of life

At the end of life when death appears imminent, the aim of care is to provide comfort, support and relief of symptoms. In these circumstances, a tube feed may be inappropriate, even though the patient is eating little.[17,18]

Patients unable to make a decision about treatment

At present in English law (there are differences in Scotland), a doctor has a duty to make decisions on behalf of an incompetent patient in their 'best interest' and in the light of previously expressed wishes by the patient, either formally as an advance directive, or informally as an expressed wish or opinion. When a decision is made to withhold or withdraw artificial nutrition, full consultation with nursing and other colleagues, and with those closest to the patient, is needed before a decision is made.[14,18] In the future, legislation may be enacted that enables a person nominated by the patient to have a continuing power of attorney

---

*Useful information is available from the Mental Health Act Commission, Maid Marion House, 56 Hounds Gate, Nottingham NG1 6BG.

with authority to make decisions about health care on his or her behalf should s/he become mentally incapacitated. Even so, decisions about withholding or withdrawing artificial nutrition will require the previous specific expressed wish of the patient.[19] The presence of dysphasia, dysarthria, and possibly limited comprehension after a stroke often make it difficult to know whether informed consent by the patient can be obtained or whether s/he is incompetent to make a decision. Every effort should be made to ascertain the patient's wishes whenever possible.

Gastrostomy feeding after a stroke

The decision to offer percutaneous endoscopic gastrostomy (PEG) feeding for stroke patients with dysphagia is often not straightforward. Many stroke patients who receive PEG tubes are severely disabled and may even be in the terminal phase of their illness, raising questions as to the appropriateness of the intervention. Factors to be considered when making such a decision are described in the section on the management of dysphagia in hospital (section 5.4).

Difficulties in decision making are related to uncertainty of prognosis, undue expectations of relatives, pressures to shorten hospital admissions, the preference of nursing homes to care for a PEG rather than a nasogastric tube, and the potential inadequacy and time-consuming nature of hand feeding.

In discussion with the patient, and those closest to him/her, the likely outcomes as regards ability to swallow and recovery of independence should be fully discussed. If it is agreed that the patient is unable to make a decision, and has not made her/his wishes known previously, the doctor should make a firm recommendation based on what appears to be the patient's best interest rather than put the responsibility of the decision on a relative. It is interesting that in future legislation an assessment of a patient's best interests is likely to include 'factors the person would consider if able to do so'.[19] It seems possible that many patients would wish to be informed about the likely impact of a particular treatment on those closest to them and would take this into account when making their decision about accepting or refusing it.

For patients who have dysphagia 2–4 weeks following stroke but with an otherwise good quality of life, physicians should undoubtedly offer PEG feeding. For those who are dying following a stroke, palliative care should be offered. The intermediate group of patients in whom there is some initial improvement but who are left with considerable disability, including dysphagia, present individual problems in management. Controlled trials comparing different methods of nutritional management after stroke are currently in progress and will provide data on which management in the future can be based.

Tube feeding of patients with advanced dementia

Another group of predominantly elderly patients who pose particular ethical and practical feeding problems are those with advanced dementia who refuse food and drink, or take only very little with much effort on the part of carers. This situation tends to occur late in the course of the illness and can be part of terminal events. The role of tube feeding for such patients is controversial in the ethical and theological literature.[20] The commonest objectives for the use of a tube feed are to prolong life and to reduce aspiration.[21] However, feeding by tube reduces mortality only by a small extent at best in patients with dementia[22,23] and aspiration may persist.[24] In one series of 103 such patients, 54% were dead within a month of introducing a gastrostomy and 90% were dead within a year.[22] Feeding tubes are poorly tolerated by demented patients and in one survey only a minority of carers felt that quality of life had been improved by the insertion of the tube.[21] Even if the aim of increasing nutritional intake is achieved, this may not result in weight gain, in contrast to PEG feeding in patients with swallowing problems secondary to other neurological diseases such as stroke and motor neurone disease. This failure to gain weight is likely to be because of the presence of cachexia-inducing cytokines.[25] It seems that in many cases refusal of food and drink, or difficulty in mastication or swallowing, is a terminal feature of the illness and good palliative care is often the most humane approach. However, the evidence is not so clear cut as to justify refusing a trial of tube feeding in all such cases on grounds of futility or risk.[20] The same principles of careful and non-directive discussions with all those involved in the care should be applied as with severely disabled stroke patients.[14]

References

1   Windsor JA, Hill GL. Weight loss with physiological impairment; a basic indicator of surgical risk. *Ann Surg* 1988; **207**: 290–6.

2   Allison SP. The uses and limitations of nutritional support. *Clin Nutr* 1992; **11**: 319–30.

3   Rayman MP. Dietary selenium: time to act. Low bioavailability in Britain and Europe could be contributing to cancers, cardiovascular disease, and subfertility. *BMJ* 1997; **314**: 387–8.

4   Council of Europe. *Partial agreement in the social and public health field. Food and nutritional care in hospitals: how to prevent undernutrition: report and guidelines.* Strasbourg: Council of Europe, 2001 (provisional edition).

5   Elia M (ed.). *Detection and management of undernutrition.* A report by the Malnutrition Advisory Group (a working group of the British Association for Parenteral and Enteral Nutrition). Maidenhead: BAPEN, 2000.

6   Corish CA, Kennedy NP. Protein-energy undernutrition in hospital in-patients: review article. *Br J Nutr* 2000; **83**: 575–91.

7   Elia M, Stratton RJ. How much undernutrition is there in hospitals? *Br J Nutr* 2000; **84**: 257–9.

8   Corish CA, Flood P, Mulligan S, Kennedy NP. Apparent low frequency of undernutrition in Dublin hospital in-patients: should we review the anthropometric thresholds for clinical practice? *Br J Nutr* 2000; **84**: 325–35.

9   UK Central Council for Nursing, Midwifery and Health Visitors. Registrar's letter sent to all nurses. London: UKCC, 1997.

10 Bond S (ed). *Eating matters.* Centre for Health Services Research, University of Newcastle upon Tyne, 1997.

11 British Dietetic Association. *Malnutrition in hospital.* Position paper. Birmingham: British Dietetic Association, 1996.

12 Audit Commission. *Acute hospital portfolio: catering, review of national findings.* Wetherby: Audit Commission Publications, 2001.

13 British Artificial Nutrition Survey (BANS). *Trends in artificial nutrition in the U.K. during 1996-2000.* Maidenhead: British Association For Parenteral and Artificial Nutrition (BAPEN), 2001.

14 Department of Health. *Reference guide to consent for examination or treatment.* London: DH, 2001.

15 British Medical Association and The Law Society. *Assessment of medical capacity: guidance for doctors and lawyers.* London: British Medical Association, 1995.

16 Mental Health Act Commission. *Guidance note 3. Guidance on the treatment of anorexia nervosa under the Mental Health Act 1983.* Nottingham: Mental Health Act Commission, 1997.

17 British Medical Association. *Withholding and withdrawing life prolonging medical treatment: guidance for decision making.* London: British Medical Association, 1999.

18 Lennard-Jones JE. Giving or withholding fluid and nutrients: ethical and legal aspects. *JR Coll Physicians Lond* 1999; **33**: 39–45.

19 Lord Chancellor's Department. *Making decisions: the government's proposals for making decisions on behalf of mentally incapacitated adults* (A report issued in the light of responses to the consultation paper, *Who Decides?*) Cm 4465. London: HMSO, 1999.

20 Gillick MR. Rethinking the role of tube feeding in patients with advanced dementia. *N Eng J Med* 2000; **342**: 206–10.

21 Mitchell S, Berkowitz RE, Lawson FME, Lipsitz LA. A cross-national survey of tube-feeding decisions in cognitively impaired older persons. *J Am Geriatr Soc* 2000; **48**: 391–7.

22 Sanders DS, Carter MJ, D'Silva J *et al.* Survival analysis in percutaneous endoscopic gastrostomy feeding: a worse outcome in patients with dementia. *Am J Gastroenterol* 2000; **95**: 1472–5.

23 Rudberg MA, Egleston BL, Grant MD, Brody JA. Effectiveness of feeding tubes in nursing home residents with swallowing disorders. *JPEN* 2000; **24**: 97–102.

24 Finucane TE, Bynum JPW. Use of tube feeding to prevent aspiration pneumonia. *Lancet* 1996; **348**: 1421–4.

25 Yeh S-S, Schuster MW. Geriatric cachexia: the role of cytokines. *Am J Clin Nutr* 1999; **70**: 183–97.

PART TWO

Community care

3 | Preventive nutritional care in the community

SUMMARY

■ During active adult life, nutritional care has the important preventive function of encouraging people to eat a balanced diet, avoiding both potentially harmful thinness and excess weight.

■ All clinical contacts give an opportunity for review of lifestyle and dietary advice if needed.

■ The potential for undernutrition among vulnerable groups should be recognised.

■ Older people who are housebound or need residential or nursing care tend to become undernourished and steps should be taken to minimise this tendency.

■ Osteoporosis is a well-known risk among older people; calcium and/or vitamin D depletion are among the many possible contributory factors.

3.1 Educational opportunities

Given the sheer size of the problem, primary health care teams alone cannot tackle the growing epidemic of obesity in the general population. UK governments have recognised the need to tackle obesity in their strategies for promoting health. The NHS and its partner organisations at local level are required to draw up health improvement plans in line with national strategic aims. For example, there is a National Service Framework aimed at reducing the mortality from coronary heart disease which necessarily includes attention to obesity, physical activity and diet.[1] The National Audit Office has issued a report on the problem of obesity and the benefits in public health likely to accrue from a decreased prevalence of obesity in the population.[2] The Faculty of Public Health Medicine of the Royal Colleges of Physicians has published a 'Toolbox'[3] for tackling obesity at local level by dietary modification and regular exercise, involving a partnership between diverse agencies such as schools (providing young people with, and educating them about, a healthy diet), industry and leisure services (providing facilities for enjoyable exercise), and the media, as well as primary health care teams at both a community and individual level.

3.2 Advice on lifestyle and diet

As the Nutrition Task Force stated, 'Primary care is an ideal setting for the opportunistic delivery of dietary advice'[4] because 70% of a practice population see their general practitioner in any year and this rises to 90% over a five-year period. Indeed, the average patient now consults a general practitioner about four times a year[5] and in addition there are consultations with practice nurses and other members of the primary care team. As the average patient remains registered with a practice for 12.7 years, there are ample opportunities to use the relationship to influence patients' lifestyles.

The public see primary care staff as credible and acceptable sources of lifestyle advice,[6] and there appears to be no lack of enthusiasm for dietary advice. The diversity of nursing roles in the primary care setting allows nurses to play a pivotal role in the promotion of good nutrition and health, including weight control, in all age groups. A South Tyneside study found that the public wanted general practitioners and practice nurses to be more involved in offering advice on lifestyle change.[7]

Primary health care teams can contribute to public education on the adverse health risks of obesity, and simple measures to avoid it, by placing 'healthy eating' posters and literature in waiting areas. A variety of such materials, based on the Government's advice in *The balance of good health*,[8] and independent of commercial sponsorship, is available from the Food Standards Agency.* *The balance of good health* has also been adapted for different ethnic groups.

Doctors and nurses in primary care can seize the opportunity to give nutritional advice when it becomes apparent during a consultation that a person is under- or overweight (see Case Study 1), in the same way that they may give advice about smoking, excess alcohol consumption or any other aspect of an unhealthy lifestyle.

3.3 Undernutrition among vulnerable groups

Even in a relatively affluent society, undernutrition is still a significant problem among certain groups of people. Primary health care teams need to target their attention towards particularly vulnerable groups (see Box 3.1).

---

*Food Standards Agency, Aviation House, 125 Kingsway, London WC2B 6NH. Tel 0845 606 0667. email: foodstandards@eclogistics.co.uk

CASE STUDY 1 – Ms T was 32 years old and in her third pregnancy. Previously she had delivered vaginally two children weighing 3.8 and 4.4 kg. In this pregnancy, the labour was prolonged and the second stage was complicated by shoulder dystocia. The mother suffered a third degree perineal tear and post-partum haemorrhage, whilst the infant had neonatal hypoglycaemia. The mother's BMI (not previously calculated, as height was not measured) was 42. Her fasting plasma glucose after pregnancy was 5.7; there was a strong family history of obesity and type II diabetes mellitus.

Comment – Maternal obesity is associated with heavy birth weight infants (even without maternal diabetes), mechanical problems at delivery and post-partum haemorrhage. It is not known whether dietary management during pregnancy can prevent these obstetric difficulties. However, if her height had been measured and BMI calculated at antenatal booking, the risk could have been predicted. She probably had gestational diabetes that would predict later type II diabetes. It is believed that dietary and exercise management following pregnancy can delay the progression to type II diabetes mellitus.

Box 3.1 Groups of people vulnerable to undernutrition

People with illness-related undernutrition
- severe disorder of any body system
- malignant disease

People in need of nutritional support before or after hospital admission
- undernutrition correctable before elective surgery
- those convalescent after major surgery or severe illness

People with difficulty in eating
- poor dentition or a sore mouth
- mastication or swallowing disorders
- sensory loss
- disorder of upper limb

Those in a vulnerable psychosocial situation
- the elderly living alone, especially after loss of a spouse
- people with learning disabilities living alone
- those affected by poverty or social isolation
- people in nursing or residential homes

People suffering from psychological illness
- depression or other mental disorders
- behavioural eating disorders

3.4 Eating disorders

As is well known, eating disorders in varying degrees of severity are common, especially among younger women, but they also occur in men. Management of these disorders often requires skilled treatment and is outside the remit of this report.

Mild anorexia (BMI = 22–18) may present with reduced food intake, an interest in being slimmer, and increased exercise. Moderate anorexia (BMI = 18–13.5) is associated with restriction of eating, withdrawal from normal relationships, amenorrhoea and family concern. Referral for specialist treatment is advisable if a patient loses more than 1 kg in weight per week or 10% of body weight over 3 months. Severe anorexia (BMI = 13.5 or below) is associated with marked psychological abnormalities, and the loss of body tissue is dangerous (see Case study 2).

CASE STUDY 2 – Miss H, aged 24, with a previous history of depression, was transferred to a psychiatric unit for investigation and management of anorexia nervosa.

On examination she was severely flat in mood, catatonic and uncooperative. She refused to eat or drink and i.v. fluid replacement therapy was commenced. It was impossible to determine how much weight she had lost recently and her BMI was estimated to be 14–15. The initial advice from the nutritional support team was that attempts should be made to feed her enterally. However, despite repeated attempts, it was not possible to intubate her with a nasogastric feeding tube. Insertion of a percutaneous endoscopic gastrostomy feeding tube was not accepted.

In view of her poor nutritional state, it was decided to institute parenteral nutritional support via a central line introduced in the arm. With careful monitoring, parenteral nutrition was successfully administered for six weeks. By the end of this time, Miss H had become more cooperative and permission was granted to insert a nasogastric feeding tube for enteral nutrition. Though the initial plan was to try to re-introduce oral nutrition, for three months this was not possible and she was fed solely via the nasogastric feeding tube by which time her BMI had increased to 16. At this stage, Miss H became cooperative enough to take some food and oral nutritional supplements. For the next month, enteral tube feeding was continued at night with oral nutrition during the day. Her psychiatric condition steadily improved and enteral tube feeding was now stopped. Throughout the remaining two months of her admission, normal food was supplemented with oral nutritional supplements and on discharge her BMI had risen to 18. Rehabilitation proceeded very satisfactorily and Miss H, who remains under the care of the psychiatrists, has been rehabilitated into the community.

Comment – This case illustrates how severe psychiatric illness can be complicated by disease-related malnutrition. This patient required parenteral nutrition initially as a life-saving measure and, as treatment progressed, she benefited from all the other forms of nutritional support, namely enteral nutrition as the sole form of nutritional intake, supplemental enteral tube feeding and finally the use of oral nutritional supplements.

Binge eating may not be associated with nutritional abnormalities, unlike compulsive overeating which can lead to a person becoming overweight or obese.

3.5 Diet of elderly people who are housebound or in residential care

It is generally recognised that the independence of older people should be preserved for as long as possible and that any period of dependence due to deterioration in physical or mental function should be as short as possible. Although basal metabolic rate falls progressively with advancing age, largely attributable to loss of muscle tissue, energy expenditure does not fall proportionately because the energy cost of normal activities such as walking may rise by as much as 20–25% due to slower speed and decreased efficiency of movement. Values (kcal/day) for daily energy intake quoted from seven studies in different countries for independent older people living in the community were 2,050–2,440 kcal daily for men and 1,600–2,100 for women.[9]

Several studies have shown that older people in long-term care tend to lose weight progressively. For older people who are dependent on others for their meals, several factors are important. Older people tend to eat little and often, to 'graze' rather than eat relatively in-frequent large meals.[10] They prefer familiar foods in small quantities at a time, whereas institutional meals are often provided two or three times a day at set times. The lack of snacks between meals and at bed-time may be a major factor contributing to a low total daily intake. Older people need adequate time to eat a meal because they often eat slowly. Meals need to be tasty, possibly with enhanced taste to com-pensate for sensory loss,[11] appropriate in consistency, attractively presented and eaten in agreeable surroundings. Some older people need special measures, such as modified cutlery or feeding utensils to compensate for physical disability, or help with opening containers, cutting up food or assistance with getting food to the mouth, and encouragement to chew and swallow.

Protein and energy intake

Detailed studies using chemical analysis of duplicate diet portions and metabolic balance studies have shown that 20 housebound older sub-jects consumed less energy-giving foods than an otherwise compara-ble group of 24 apparently healthy older people. The mean energy intake of the housebound group was approximately one-third lower than of the apparently healthy subjects, and 12 out of 20 had energy intakes lower than their calculated resting metabolic rate.[12] Attention to energy intake is therefore appropriate for housebound subjects, as for those in residential care.

The healthy subjects were in overall nitrogen balance with a mean protein intake equivalent to 0.97 g/kg body weight per day, whereas the housebound subjects ate less protein and were in negative balance for nitrogen with a mean protein intake equivalent to 0.67 g/kg body weight per day.[12] A longitudinal study over 10 years among free-living older persons has shown that those who consumed at least 1 g of protein per kg body weight daily had a lower mortality than those who consumed less protein.[13] It seems advisable therefore to aim for an intake of approximately 1 g of protein per kg body weight daily for older people.

Fruit, vegetables and cereals

A balance has to be struck between the need for small, frequent, energy-rich meals and snacks, an adequate fibre intake to maintain bowel function, and fruit and fresh vegetables to provide vitamin C.

Minerals, trace elements and vitamin

Balance data show that apparently healthy older people were in calcium balance while taking 1 g of calcium daily, whereas housebound people were in negative balance taking 0.8 g of calcium daily. These results are in line with data from therapeutic trials discussed below. Balance studies for zinc, copper, iron, manganese, chromium and selenium showed that housebound subjects differed significantly from healthy subjects only in negative zinc and copper balance.[12]

3.6 Increasing the nutritional intake of elderly people in residential care

First, the tendency of such people to lose weight must be recognised by all responsible for their care. Those people who enter residential care in an undernourished state are at particular risk of further weight loss and their condition must be identified on admission. However, even those without evidence of prior undernutrition also tend to lose weight when they are dependent on institutional care (see Table 1.2).[14] A system of regular monitoring of food intake, meals uneaten or only partially eaten, and body weight should be standard practice.

Each person requires individual assessment. There may be a medical and remediable reason for poor appetite, such as a drug side-effect, sore mouth or infection.[10] The patient may need special attention at meals because of a physical disability such as poor sight, muscular weakness due to a stroke or other cause, or mental impairment. Attention is needed to all the general factors related to meals described above.

A controlled therapeutic trial involving 501 patients in a Swedish residential care home has shown that giving a liquid nutritional supplement in addition to the regular diet, decreased subsequent mortality[14] and this effect was noted among both subjects who appeared normally nourished and those who were undernourished on admission. Thus there is justification for use of such supplements, which include micronutrients, if weight cannot be maintained by means of an energy-rich diet and snacks of ordinary food.

3.7 Nutritional aspects of osteoporosis

Osteoporosis is common in an ageing population. It has been estimated that the lifetime risk of bone fracture among white women at the time of the menopause is 30–40% and the risk for a man aged 50 is approximately one-fifth of these figures.[15] Prevention (increase in bone density) and treatment (prevention of fracture) involve lifestyle and hormonal or drug regimens which have been well reviewed and guidelines prepared.[15,16] This report deals solely with the nutritional aspects of osteoporosis.

There is epidemiological evidence that very thin women are at increased risk of fractured hip. A cohort of 3,595 white women aged 40–77 years was followed for an average of 10 years during which 84 new hip fractures were identified. There was a strong correlation between this risk and a low body mass index, a small cross-sectional area of arm muscle or thin triceps skin fold. People who were active in recreation were at reduced risk of fracture.[17] Three possible factors have been suggested to account for the relationship between muscle mass, subcutaneous fat and bone fracture. The force that muscle exerts on bone could be a trophic factor; muscle and fat may also cushion the bone during a fall. There is also the possibility that undernutrition affects both muscle and bone mass, leading to weak muscles and fragile bone.

The role of low calcium and/or vitamin D intake as factors in loss of bone mass, in addition to the effects of low oestrogen levels, smoking and age, is unclear. Vitamin D stimulates calcium absorption by the gut and its effect is particularly important when calcium intake is marginal; when calcium intake is high, passive absorption is more important.[18] The recommended dietary intake of calcium for adults and elderly people is 700 mg per day. The major source is milk, and milk products. Between 1975 and 1990 the mean total milk and cream consumed by older people declined from 5.57 to 4.3 pints per week.[9]

The predominant source of vitamin D is from ultraviolet irradiation of the skin by sunlight of a wavelength which occurs in the UK between May and September. Food provides small amounts of vitamin D, principally in fatty fish, eggs, liver, butter and fortified margarine or cereals.[9] It has been estimated that the mean dietary intake of vitamin D is approximately 2 µg/day. In the absence of cutaneous synthesis, an intake of 5–10 µg/day is required to ensure plasma levels above those associated with osteomalacia.[9] The recommended daily intake of vitamin D is 10 µg/day.[9] Surveys have shown that serum 25-hydoxyvitamin D concentration was frequently low among older people living in retirement or nursing homes in Europe, and among hospital inpatients in the USA.[19]

Since there is a potential deficiency of both dietary calcium and vitamin D in older people, the results of controlled trials of supplementation are instructive.[15] For example, in France, 3,270 women aged 69–106 years of age living in nursing homes or apartment houses for elderly people were studied.[20] Half took 1.2 g of elemental calcium and 20 µg (800 IU) of vitamin D daily for 18 months and the other half took control preparations. The estimated daily calcium intake in both groups at onset was approximately 500 mg daily. On an intention-to-treat basis, there were 160 non-vertebral fractures in the active group and 215 in the control group ($p < 0.001$); these included 80 and 110 hip fractures respectively ($p = 0.004$). The bone density of the proximal femoral region increased by 2.7% in the active group and decreased by 4.6% in the control group ($p < 0.001$).

A similar trial was conducted in the eastern USA among 430 people of both sexes, all aged at least 65 years and living in the community.[21] The active treatment group took tablets containing 500 mg of elemental calcium and 17.5 µg (700 IU) of vitamin D daily for 3 years. There were 11 non-vertebral fractures among these subjects compared with 26 among those who took placebo tablets ($p = 0.02$). Measurements showed increases in mineral density of the femoral neck ($p = 0.02$) and total body ($p = <0.001$) in the 148 people who completed 3 years treatment whereas there were decreases in these measurements among 170 control subjects over the same period.

Calcium supplementation of 1 g daily, without vitamin D, over 4 years among 38 younger post-menopausal women resulted in reduced bone loss and fewer fractures than among 40 matched subjects who took a control tablet.[22] It is not possible from the published trials to determine whether the addition of vitamin D in physiological doses to a calcium supplement is beneficial.[15]

Guidelines based on these and other trials suggest that there is good evidence for giving a calcium and vitamin D supplement to frail elderly people with increased risk of falling, whether or not they are confined indoors.[16] This recommendation is supported by recent reviews which extend the recommendations to all elderly people and others at risk.[18,19,23] Vitamin D and calcium are generally regarded as adjuncts to hormonal or drug treatment or drug treatment for established osteoporosis.[16]

References

1 Department of Health. *National Service Framework for Coronary Heart Disease: modern standards and service models.* London: DH, 2000.

2 National Audit Office. *Tackling obesity in England.* London: The Stationery Office, 2001.

3 Maryon Davis A, Giles A, Rona R. *Tackling obesity: a toolbox for local partnership action.* London: Faculty of Public Health Medicine of the Royal Colleges of Physicians of the UK, 2000.

4 Department of Health. *Eat well. An action plan from the Nutrition Task Force to achieve the Health of the Nation targets on diet and nutrition.* London: DH, 1994.

5 Office of Populations, Censuses and Surveys, Royal College of General Practitioners, and Department of Health. *Morbidity statistics from general practice. Fourth national study 1991–1992.* London: HMSO, 1995.

6 Buttriss JL. Food and nutrition: attitudes, beliefs and knowledge in the United Kingdom. *Am J Clin Nutr* 1997; **65**(suppl): 1985s–1995s.

7 Gallagher M. Patients' views. *Practice Nursing,* 8 March, p.15.

8 Department of Health. *The balance of good health.* Middlesex: Food Standards Agency.

9 Working Group on the Nutrition of Elderly People of the Committee on Medical Aspects of Food Policy. *The nutrition of elderly people.* Department of Health Report on Health and Social Subjects, 43. London: HMSO, 1992.

10 Allison SP. Cost-effectiveness of nutritional support in the elderly. *Proc Nutr Soc* 1995; **54**: 693–9.

11 Schiffman SS. Taste and smell losses in normal ageing and disease. *JAMA* 1997; **278**: 1357–62.

12 Bunker VW, Clayton BE. Research review: studies in the nutrition of elderly people with particular reference to essential trace elements. *Age Ageing* 1989; **18**: 422–9.

13 Vellas BJ, Hunt WC, Romero LJ *et al.* Changes in nutritional status and patterns of morbidity among free-living elderly persons: a 10-year longitudinal study. *Nutrition* 1997; **13**: 515–19.

14 Larsson J, Unosson M, Ek A-C *et al.* Effect of dietary supplement on nutritional status and clinical outcome in 501 geriatric patients (a randomized study). *Clin Nutr* 1990; **9**: 179–84.

15 Royal College of Physicians. *Osteoporosis: clinical guidelines for prevention and treatment.* London: RCP, 1999.

16 Royal College of Physicians and Bone and Tooth Society of Great Britain. *Osteoporosis: clinical guidelines for prevention and treatment. Update on pharmacological interventions and an algorithm for management.* London: RCP, 2000.

17 Farmer ME, Harris T, Madans JH *et al.* Anthropometric indicators and hip fracture: the NHANES 1 epidemiologic follow-up study. *J Am Geriatr Soc* 1989; **37**: 9–16.

18 Prince RL. Diet and the prevention of osteoporotic fractures. *N Engl J Med* 1997; **337**: 701–2.

19 Utiger RD. The need for more vitamin D. *N Engl J Med* 1998; **338**: 828–9.
20 Chapuy MC, Arlot ME, Duboeuf F *et al.* Vitamin D3 and calcium to prevent hip fractures in elderly women. *N Engl J Med* 1992; **327**: 1637–42.
21 Dawson-Hughes B, Harris SS, Krall EA, Dallal GE. Effect of calcium and vitamin D supplementation on bone density in men and women 65 years of age or older. *N Engl J Med* 1997; **337**: 670–6.
22 Reid IR, Ames RW, Evans MC *et al.* Long-term effects of calcium supplementation on bone loss and fractures in postmenopausal women: a randomized controlled trial. *Am J Med* 1995; **98**: 331–5.
23 Compston JE. Vitamin D deficiency: time for action. Evidence supports routine supplementation for elderly people and others at risk. *BMJ* 1998; **317**: 1466–7.

4 | Therapeutic nutritional care in the community

SUMMARY

- Once undernutrition or obesity is recognised, positive steps can be taken to remedy the situation.
- Undernutrition may necessitate attention to food intake and sometimes the use of dietary supplements.
- The number of patients being discharged from hospital to continue a tube feed in the community is increasing. Close liaison between hospital and primary care teams is essential.
- A practice register of obese patients who would derive clinical benefit from weight reduction is recommended.
- Clinical intervention that aims to help obese patients achieve weight reduction of 5-10% is realistic and clinicaly beneficial, but is time consuming and requires organisation.

4.1 Management of undernutrition

Food

For those who cannot obtain good food for any reason, increasing its availability is usually the first line of treatment. Assistance with shopping, cooking, or eating may therefore be needed. Referral to a community dietitian can be helpful, and social services and voluntary organisations such as Meals on Wheels can be mobilised to help improve a patient's diet. Day centres, day hospitals and lunch clubs also provide nutritious meals. Help the Aged and Age Concern produce leaflets about nutrition geared for the elderly. For those who have little appetite because they are ill, special meals may be needed. Those who are averse to eating for psychological reasons may be helped by psychiatric treatments.

Supplements

If it is not possible to meet nutritional requirements from food, a liquid medicinal supplement can be prescribed to give an additional intake of 300–600 kcal (1–2 cartons) daily. The flavour and texture of the supplement must be acceptable to the patient, who also needs advice on the best way to take it. The use of supplements has increased even more in

41

CASE STUDY 3 – Mr J, aged 62, with a known history of chronic obstructive pulmonary disease (COPD), consulted his general practitioner who diagnosed acute bronchitis and prescribed antibiotics. The doctor noted, on weighing the patient, that he had lost 2 kg in the previous month and that his BMI had fallen to 18. No specific cause was found for the weight loss. An oral nutritional supplement was prescribed after dietary assessment by the community dietitian who recommended that three 200 ml cartons (900 kcal) be consumed throughout the day in addition to the patient's normal diet. Mr J was assessed at monthly intervals by the dietitian and at the end of three months had gained 3.5 kg in weight. He said that he felt better, was less breathless and could walk longer distances. The supplements were stopped at this point.

Comment – Oral nutritional supplements are currently being prescribed more widely in the community. Their use has been associated with weight gain in a number of specific conditions including patients with COPD, among whom functional benefits include improved respiratory muscle strength, hand-grip strength and walking distance. Weight gain has been shown to be greater in adult patients with BMI <20 compared to those with a mean BMI >20. It is unclear whether the weight gain is achieved at the expense of eating normal food and most studies show that actual intake from oral nutritional supplements is less than the amount prescribed. Stopping supplements typically results in reduced total energy intake causing a loss of gained weight. The temporary benefits of oral nutritional supplements in patients with COPD are illustrated in this case study.

the community than in hospital.[1] A systematic review has identified 57 controlled trials, but in only 28 was significant weight gain observed compared with a control group.[1] In a recent National Diet and Nutrition Survey among subjects aged 65 and over,[2] about a third of those living in the community and 8% of those in institutions were taking non-prescribed supplements.

4.2 Artificial nutrition

More and more patients are being treated by artificial nutrition in the community. It is important to realise that whilst these treatments are usually beneficial, they are also associated with a risk of complications, particularly parenteral nutrition. A treatment goal is desirable for these treatments. If the ability to swallow returns or intestinal absorption improves it may be possible to stop the treatment. If the treatment fails or is burdensome, the regimen should be reviewed and appropriate changes made, including if necessary reversion to oral feeding.

Enteral tube feeding

In the year 2000, approximately 15,000 adults and 5,000 children were receiving an enteral tube feed in the community, mainly via a gastrostomy inserted in hospital by an endoscopic technique (percu-taneous endoscopic gastrostomy (PEG)) and the trend over the previous five years showed that these numbers had been increasingly steadily. Although some of these patients are managed at home by their family or carers, many are cared for in nursing homes.[3] While the primary care team may assume much of the responsibility for these patients, there should be clear care plans agreed with the hospital team, including regular expert review of the treatment and its continuing necessity. There should also be easy access to the hospital team for advice and help in the event of problems, for example a blocked or damaged feeding tube. A climate of helpful and close collaboration between all concerned is important.

Parenteral nutrition

There are also more than 500 patients who administer parenteral nutri-tion to themselves in the community, some of whom depend on the help of a carer.[3] These patients are trained in this task by the hospital nutrition team. In contrast to enteral feeding, parenteral feeding in the community will continue to be the main responsibility of the hospital expert group. It is unreasonable to expect any primary care team to supervise this highly technical treatment which is comparable to home dialysis, for example. The service may be supported by a commercial home care company suitably staffed by nurses experienced in the field. There also needs to be 'hot line' access to the hospital team so that any problems can be dealt with swiftly and expertly. The primary care team needs to understand the principles of parenteral nutrition and may assume responsibility for other aspects of the patient's care. As with enteral feeding, good communication and close collaboration between the primary and hospital care teams are needed. A clear written contract between the two is desirable, similar to those established by renal units for renal replacement therapy at home.

4.3 Overnutrition: obesity

Primary care practices are encouraged to identify those patients most likely to benefit from weight management and to set up and maintain a register of these patients with systematic records of BMI and waist circumference. Categories of such patients recommended for inclu-sion are overweight patients with non-insulin-dependent diabetes, obese patients with existing coronary heart disease, transient ischaemic attacks, high blood pressure, raised cholesterol, sleep apnoea, arthritis and back pain, and smokers.[4]

CASE STUDY 4 – Mr M, aged 45, was admitted with an acute subendocardial myocardial infarction. This was not complicated by rhythm disturbance or major left ventricular dysfunction. He was treated with thrombolysis, and later aspirin and beta-blockade. Within a year of his myocardial infraction, he was treated with a lipid-lowering agent and hypotensive therapy. It was also decided that he should have coronary artery bypass grafting. Three years after his original presentation it was felt he had impaired glucose tolerance but not diabetes. Five years after his original presentation he did present with osmotic symptoms and was diagnosed as having diabetes mellitus. This was the first time that his BMI (37) featured in his medical records. He had had four admissions to hospital and many outpatient visits since his original presentation. His weight, glycaemic control, blood pressure control and dyslipidaemia all improved, although were not cured, by a relatively modest weight loss of 4.5 kg.

Comment – Although the progress of his ischaemic heart disease could not have been prevented, it almost certainly could have been delayed by adequate nutritional screening assessment and management when he first presented. Some form of nutritional assessment should feature in the medical records whenever a patient is first seen or is re-assessed.

All such people should be offered entry into a weight loss and weight maintenance programme. The first phase will concentrate on weight loss and will usually last about 12 weeks; thereafter the emphasis will move to weight maintenance. The aim should be to achieve and sustain a 5–10% weight loss so as to improve a person's risk profile (see Fig 4). This is a goal which for many is both achievable and sustainable, unlike

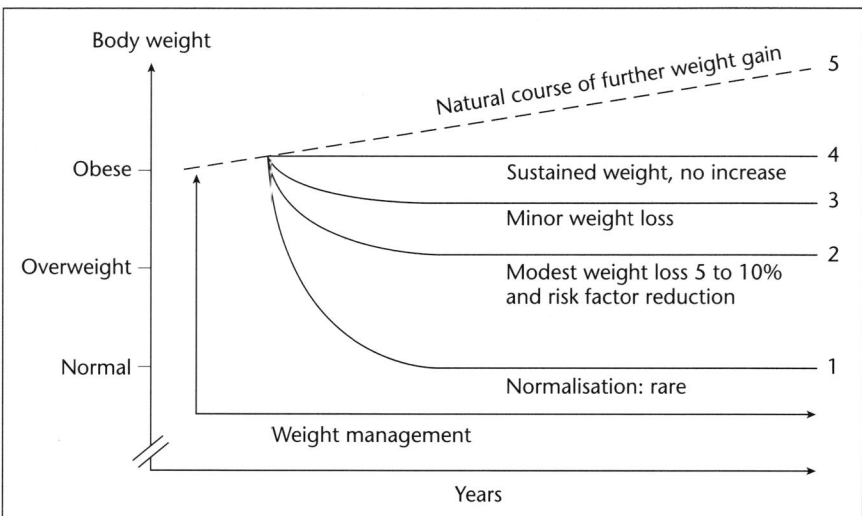

Figure 4 Realistic weight goals. The figure illustrates the possible clinical outcomes from weight management over a period of years and confirms that modest weight reduction represents an achievable goal for a patient. Adapted from Ref 5.

ideal body weight, and can have a major impact in reducing the mortality and morbidity associated with obesity. A dietary programme involving gradual weight loss through a balanced calorie-deficit diet is more likely to lead to sustained improvement (see Fig 5) than a very low calorie diet.

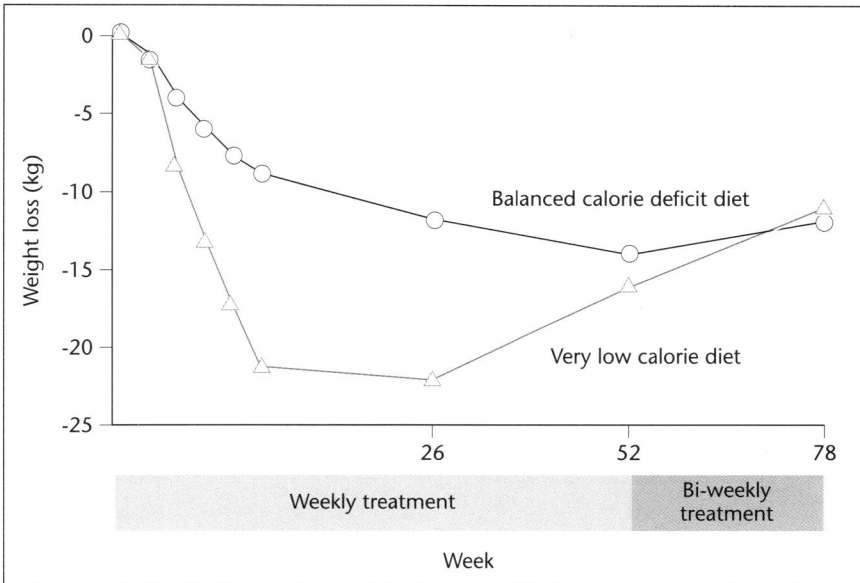

Figure 5 The weight loss achieved following two supervised dietary regimens – a balanced calorie deficit diet and a very low calorie diet. The figure confirms the frequent clinical observation of 'rebound' weight gain following an extremely restricted diet despite continuing supervision. Adapted from Ref 6.

Lifestyle advice for such patients should include both dietary change and an increase in physical activity. The benefits of physical activity are greatest in those who are habitually inactive and can be achieved by 20–30 minutes of brisk walking daily. Anti-obesity medication can be considered when appropriate, details of which are given in an RCP report.[7]

Ways of approaching the management of obesity within a community, involving the resources of primary, secondary and tertiary care, are shown in Fig 6.

Running a weight loss and weight maintenance clinic is very time consuming and there are areas where the workload of primary healthcare teams precludes them from providing the structured support and follow-up so necessary for obese people. In these circumstances, primary care trusts should consider developing weight management clinics and links with approved private organisations that offer education and group sessions to encourage weight control.

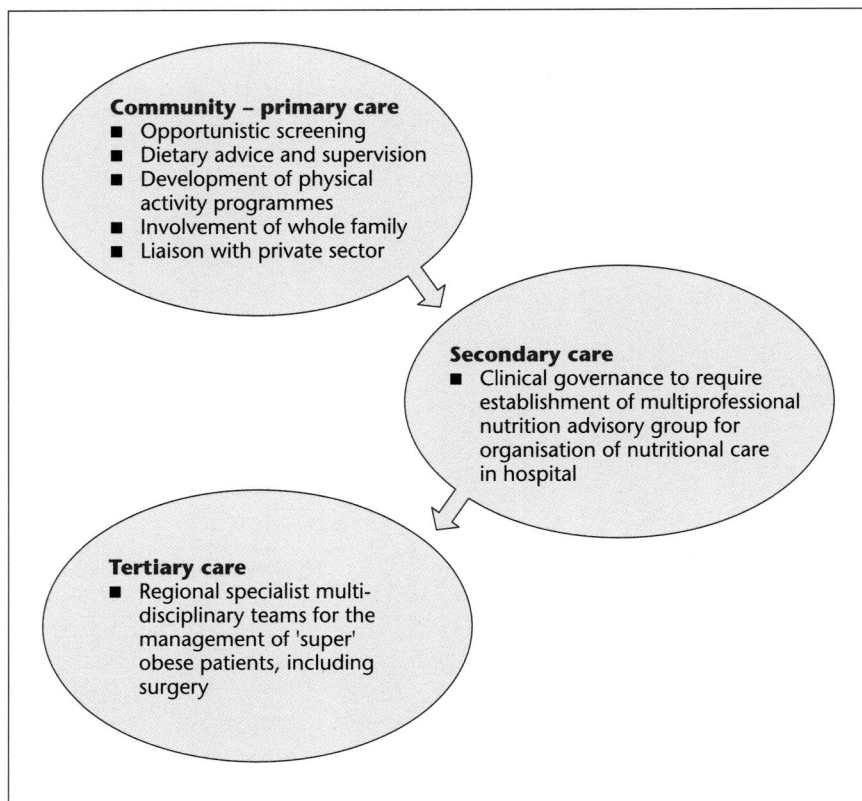

Figure 6 A possible management pathway for obesity involving primary, secondary and tertiary care.

References

1   Stratton RJ, Elia M. A critical, systematic analysis of the use of oral nutrition supplements in the community. *Clin Nutr* 1999; **18**(suppl 2): 29–84.

2   Finch S, Doyle W, Lowe C *et al. National Diet and Nutrition Survey: people aged 65 years and over. Volume 1: Report of the diet and nutrition survey.* London: The Stationery Office, 1998.

3   British Artificial Nutrition Survey (BANS). *Trends in artificial nutrition in the U.K. during 1996-2000.* Maidenhead: British Association for Parenteral and Artificial Nutrition (BAPEN), 2001.

4   Maryon Davis A, Giles A, Rona R. *Tackling obesity: a toolbox for local partnership action.* London: Faculty of Public Health Medicine of the Royal Colleges of Physicians of the UK, 2000.

5   Rössner S. Is obesity incurable? In Ditschumeit H, Gries FA, Haumer H *et al* (eds). *Obesity in Europe.* London: John Libbey & Co, 1993: 203–8.

6   Wadden TA, Foster GD, Letizia KA. One-year behavioral treatment of obesity: comparison of moderate and severe calorific restriction and the effects of weight maintenance therapy. *J Consult Clin Psychol* 1994; **62**(1): 165–71.

7   Royal College of Physicians. *Clinical management of overweight and obese patients, with particular reference to the use of drugs.* Report of a working party. London: RCP, 1998.

PART THREE

Hospital care

5 | Nutritional care in hospital

SUMMARY

- Nutritional care in hospital tends to be forgotten due to the focus on the main reason for investigation or treatment.
- Simple measures to indicate a patient's nutritional state should be recorded at every hospital consultation. Information about nutritional state should form a mandatory part of the admission record prepared by a doctor when a patient is admitted to hospital.
- Doctors need to collaborate with colleagues in other disciplines when a care plan is made to prevent or reverse under- or overnutrition, and in arrangements to monitor its outcome.
- Doctors need to appreciate the importance of dietary intake and be aware of the particular nutritional needs of elderly patients.
- Patients with difficulty in swallowing need skilled assessment and treatment.
- The use of dietary supplements requires good organisation.
- Protocols are needed to define the indications for, and implementation of, nasogastric and gastrostomy tube feeds, and parenteral nutrition.
- Doctors with a special interest in nutrition should be actively involved in a hospital nutrition support team responsible for artificial nutrition and act as a member of a nutritional steering committee responsible for policy in an NHS trust.

A patient in hospital tends to be cared for by several health care workers in different disciplines. Responsibility for nutritional care therefore tends to be fragmented unless it is well organised. Ultimate clinical responsibility lies with the doctor who needs to integrate nutritional care into basic clinical practice.

5.1 Outpatient consultation

Besides the primary reason for the consultation, meeting each patient provides an opportunity to review general health and lifestyle. All patients in a medical clinic should be weighed as part of the same routine as checking the blood pressure and the urine. If height can be recorded once as part of the basic data for a new patient, the BMI can thereafter be noted at each attendance. A glance at this figure, in conjunction with a visual impression of body build, girth, subcutaneous fat, muscle bulk and any clinical manifestations of specific deficiencies, should provide a rapid guide as to whether any nutritional advice or other action is needed. In those who are overweight, measurement of abdominal girth can be a guide to the risk of coronary heart disease and type II diabetes. Over- and undernutrition are relevant to every medical specialty, not only diabetes and metabolism.

5.2 Inpatient care

Nutritional data in the initial medical record

A doctor's initial entry in the medical record should contain a note about the patient's nutritional state. When possible, the patient should be asked about appetite, any unintended recent weight change and, if so, its magnitude (in terms of percentage of usual weight). If clinically feasible, the weight and height should be recorded; if need be, the patient's statement about height may be used. When these measurements are available, it should become routine for the BMI to be noted. In all patients, a comment should be made as to whether their nutritional state appears normal, overweight or undernourished. This may be the only note possible in those with whom communication is impossible or who cannot be weighed. A visual impression of chronic undernutrition which includes qualitative observation of subcutaneous fat, peripheral muscle bulk and any evidence of specific nutrient deficiency correlates well with anthropometric and laboratory measurements.[1,2] Hand-grip weakness and weak pulmonary expiratory force shown by an inability to cough vigorously on request, in association with recent weight loss, can be indicators of acute nutritional deprivation.[3]

Nutritional screening and assessment

Ideally, the elements of the screening tool should be scored numerically and linked to an appropriate and agreed plan of action, depending on the risk score and the clinical circumstances. The action may involve:

- observation only
- simple nursing measures such as help with eating
- referral to a dietitian, specialist clinician, speech therapist, or nutrition care team who will undertake more detailed nutritional assessment and treatment.

A National Audit Commission survey in the years 1999/2000 in England and Wales showed that in 77% of acute hospital trusts a nutritional screening protocol is in place that is carried out by nurses, but in the remainder it was not clear how patients' nutritional needs are routinely identified.[4] Doctors need to be aware of the result of nutritional screening when it indicates that a patient is under- or over-nourished, or is likely to eat little due to the illness or its treatment, and of the action proposed. Doctors should also ensure that a nutritional care plan for such a patient is recorded in the notes and that information is passed on to other doctors who may be involved in the care of the patient.

Care plan and monitoring

A nutritional care plan devised in the light of screening or assessment should be relevant to the individual patient's needs and be seen as an integral part of the patient's overall management. The doctor is in a unique position to ensure this.

While on an acute ward, a patient's nutritional status should be monitored weekly by weighing and completion of a screening tool where one is in use. The Audit Commission's survey showed that in only less than half of acute hospital trusts was patients' nutrition reviewed weekly to ensure that care was adjusted to their changing needs while in hospital.[4] The nutritional status of patients in long-stay wards should also be re-assessed regularly but usually at less frequent intervals.

The ward round

During the ward round members of the medical team not only have direct contact with the patient but also the opportunity for consultation with nursing, dietetic and other colleagues. It is customary for the team to look at the temperature and fluid balance charts, but body weight and ideally BMI should also be noted as a matter of routine, along with the result of weekly monitoring of nutritional state, including a check on whether the patient is eating and how much. If nutritional support or dietary advice is needed, the action already taken can be reported, or future policy can be agreed, and recorded in the clinical notes.

Doctors' contribution to the provision of hospital food

Unless there are contrary medical indications, ensuring that patients are adequately nourished is best achieved through the provision of hospital food (see Chapter 6), with supplements as appropriate, rather than through enteral or parenteral nutrition. Hospital meals are the most cost-effective solution (food at 2001 prices costs approximately £2.60 per day; enteral nutrition £10.00 per day; and parenteral £80.00 per day), as well as having a number of psychological and physiological advantages. It should also be remembered that food is the only complete form of nutritional support. A survey has shown that approximately 95% of patients rely on hospital food.[5]

Guidelines for hospital catering, produced as part of the Health of the Nation initiative, estimated the dietary requirements of hospital patients from the dietary reference values in health recommended by the Committee on Medical Aspects of Food Policy (COMA) of the Department of Health.[6] The guidelines suggested that hospital menus should be capable of delivering a daily range of energy intake of 1,200–2,500 kcal, with a minimum of 300 kcal for each main meal and a minimum of 500 kcal for an energy dense choice, and of 18 g of protein at each main meal. For most patients, an energy intake within the range 1,800–2,200 kcal, and a protein intake for adults of 45–55 g, were recommended.[7] A review of measurements of energy expenditure and nitrogen balance in hospital patients has concluded that these recommendations are low for some patients and that a daily intake of 30 kcal of energy and 1–1.5 g of protein for each kilogram of body weight meet the needs of the majority.[8]

Consumption of hospital food Surveys have shown that approximately 40% of food supplied to hospital wards can be wasted, either as trays of food not used or as food left on plates.[8,9,10] The Audit Commission surveyed six wards in almost every trust and found that more than three-quarters of trusts waste over 10% of the meals produced, either because the catering department issues more meals than are requested or the wards order more meals than there are patients available to eat them.[4] Plate waste in another study of four wards in one hospital amounted to 32–41%.[9] If food is uneaten, patients receive less than their minimal requirement and lose weight.[11,12] If patients become undernourished in hospital, or pre-existing undernourishment becomes worse, these are matters of clinical[13,14] and economic[15] importance.

The aim of hospital catering is to give patients a choice of appetising meals, served attractively, and eaten, with assistance if necessary, in as pleasant an environment as possible. As described in Chapter 6, there are many problems to be overcome in achieving these aims. Doctors should support all types of staff engaged in trying to provide a good service. Although the realities often fall short of the ideal, constructive encouragement helps both patients and staff.

Doctors can help to promote more satisfactory nutrition for patients by making sure that as far as possible:

■ The service and consumption of meals is not interrupted by ward rounds or routine tasks which could take place at other times.

■ Procedures, such as x-rays, are scheduled to ensure, whenever possible, that patients do not miss meals. Where this is unavoidable, or the patient's return to the ward is delayed, a meal should be available. Similarly, arrangements should be in place for when patients are away from the ward and unable to order their own food.

■ When an operation or other procedure is delayed, systems should be in place to ensure that the patient is provided with meals up to the time when nil by mouth becomes necessary again. Provision of nutrients during the peri-operative period, when early resumption of oral feeding appears to be clinically beneficial,[16] should be included in treatment plans.

Discharge from hospital

Continuity between secondary and primary care is essential and any nutritional problem that requires action or follow-up on leaving hospital should be mentioned in a hospital discharge letter. Return to a normal nutritional state will take place gradually over months after a severe illness associated with loss of several kilograms in weight. Medical supervision during convalescence can be helpful in these circumstances, as mentioned above in connection with primary care (see section 3.3).

Artificial feeding If a patient is discharged with a tube in place to continue nutritional support outside hospital, the hospital team must establish liaison with subsequent carers to make sure that they understand how to manage the nutritional support and to whom they should turn if a complication occurs. It is also essential that a firm arrangement is made for a health worker to check on the patient's progress at regular intervals, as the regime may need to be changed. For example, it may be possible to stop an enteral tube feed if the ability to swallow improves, or parenteral feeds may be reduced or stopped if intestinal absorption returns sufficiently for the patient to maintain health with oral nutrients.

5.3 Nutritional care of older patients in hospital

Approximately half of all hospital admissions are patients aged over 65 years. In a study of hospital admissions in Dundee, 43% of those admitted to medical wards for older patients were undernourished, of whom

19% were severely undernourished (BMI <16 and a triceps skinfold thickness or mid-arm circumference below the fifth centile of a reference population), and 30% were overnourished by the criteria of the National Diet and Nutrition Survey.[12,17] A review of other surveys has confirmed that malnutrition is common at the time of hospital admission, though at a somewhat lower incidence.[18,19] Severe undernutrition was observed in 138 of 744 older women admitted with fractured femur in Nottingham. Mortality was highest in this most undernourished group and the survivors took longer to rehabilitate than the better nourished.[20,21] The Committee on Medical Aspects of Food Policy[6] recommended that reference values for protein, non-starch polysaccharides and micronutrients should be the same for younger and older persons and these values have been accepted as the standard in *Nutrition guidelines for hospital catering.*[7]

Energy and protein

A study has shown that patients in two UK acute hospital wards for older people took an average of 1,379 kcal and 44.6 g of protein daily as compared with a maximum provision in the hospital meals of 2,438 kcal and 67 g of protein. Wastage of food at main meals by waste on plates averaged 42%.[9] A detailed study by chemical analysis of duplicate food portions among 21 older patients in a long-stay ward showed a mean intake of metabolisable energy of 1,229 kcal and of 44.6 g of protein (0.79 g/kg body weight) daily. These levels were one-third and one-quarter respectively lower than for a control group of apparently healthy elderly subjects living at home.[22] During one year of observation, weight losses of 2–6 kg were observed in 13 of these 21 patients.

Three studies have shown that increasing the energy content of meals by adding fat, oils or carbohydrate results in a higher intake. In a Swedish study, foods providing meals fortified with high-energy constituents, but of unchanged volume, resulted in an increase of average energy consumption from 1,350 kcal/day to 1,825 kcal/day.[23] In a British study, such a policy increased energy intake by approximately 20% among older subjects in hospital.[24] In a second British study, not only was the energy content of meals increased but the portion size was reduced, resulting in a mean rise of energy consumption at the two main meals from 1,425 to 1,711 kcal daily and a reduction in plate waste from 42 to 27%.[25] These findings emphasise the need of older people in hospital for energy dense meals which contain a higher proportion of fat and sugar than is recommended for healthy adults in younger age groups. Older people also cope better with smaller portions at each meal.

Besides a different energy density of main meals, older people also require frequent snacks between meals or food supplements. Snacks can take the form of cakes, biscuits, sandwiches and nutritious drinks. Alternatively, or in addition, a liquid or semi-solid medicinal nutritional supplement can be given. A controlled trial in hospital among patients with an average age of approximately 70 years has shown that by prescribing a liquid supplement it was possible to increase daily energy intake to 1,680 kcal as compared with 1,250 kcal in a control group.[26] The mean duration of the trial was 8.9 days in the control group and 9.7 days among those who received supplements; a mean weight loss of 2.5% occurred among the former and a gain of 2.9% among the latter.

Fibre

If meal size is to be kept small for older people, but with a high energy content, it may be difficult to include adequate fresh vegetables, fruit and other non-starch polysaccharides. Older people tend to suffer from constipation so adequate fibre is important, though a bran supplement can lead to loose stools and incontinence.[27]

Minerals, trace elements and vitamins

The rationale for a supplement of vitamin D, and possibly calcium, for older people in general has been discussed above (section 3.7). A detailed study in a geriatric unit of three wards, based on weighed food intake and composition tables, showed that the mean intake of calcium was approximately 800 mg daily, largely contributed by milk. Intake of vitamins A and D tended to be low. Vitamin C intake calculated from food tables appeared to be adequate but when duplicate food portions were analysed chemically much lower intakes were found as a result of food processing.[28] A case can therefore be made for giving a regular multivitamin tablet to older long-stay patients.

Zinc and copper intake has been analysed chemically in food portions of long-stay patients in wards for the elderly and found to be low. However, among these patients there was no correlation between zinc and copper levels in the blood and poor healing of leg ulcers or pressure sores.[22]

5.4 Nutritional care of patients with difficulty in swallowing

Difficulty in swallowing (dysphagia) can be due to infections involving the mouth or pharynx, weakness or inco-ordination of the swallowing mechanism, or obstruction. The latter can often be overcome by giving nutrient liquid feeds or by tube feeding. The commonest form of neurological dysphagia is a stroke.

Nutritional care after a stroke

Undernutrition on admission to hospital after a stroke is a strong and independent predictor of morbidity and mortality.[29] Oral nutritional support given acutely and extended during the rehabilitation phase has been found to improve the nutritional status of stroke patients[30] but it is not known whether this improves the clinical outcome. A large multicentre trial is in progress designed to answer this question. However, the nutritional needs of stroke patients are often unrecognised, especially during the rehabilitation phase when independent feeding is resumed and energy requirements go up but energy and protein intakes may be lower than when assisted feeding is needed.[28]

Early assessment of capacity to swallow when there is doubt about this function must be regarded as an integral part of the team approach to the management of stroke patients at risk. At present, a decision about the ability of a patient to take normal, semi-solid or liquid nutrients by mouth tends to await assessment of dysphagia by a speech and language therapist. This practice may lead to delay as these specialists are relatively few in number. Their function is to advise the doctor in charge who will make the decision. Some nurses are being trained by speech and language therapists to assess ability to swallow as an extension of their Scope of Professional Practice but the number of nurses so trained is small. As most doctors have to care for patients with neurological disability at some stage in their career, it seems important that undergraduates, and postgraduates when appropriate, should be taught how to assess clinical dysphagia by simple clinical criteria as part of their basic training.

The indications for, and role of, tube feeding can be considered in two phases: immediate treatment and the possible need for long-term tube feeding in the community. Most patients who are dysphagic immediately after a stroke recover the ability to swallow. In a series of 357 patients, conscious after hemispheric stroke and assessed within 48 hours, one-third were dysphagic. Half recovered the ability to swallow within one week and only 2% of survivors were still dysphagic at one month.[31] This figure is consistent with an estimate that approximately 1.7% of all patients in the UK who suffered a stroke in 1998 were discharged from hospital to continue tube feeding in the community.[32] A good case can therefore be made for persisting with nasogastric feeding when possible for at least two weeks and if possible for longer, in the hope that swallowing ability will return.

PEG after stroke: what you should consider

The following facts are relevant when considering the insertion of a PEG for a patient after a stroke:

- Placement of a PEG tube is not without risk, and death within a few days may occur if inappropriate high-risk patients are selected.[33] If the patient's cardio-respiratory state is poor, or for any other reason death within a month appears likely, then a PEG is contra-indicated.

- Insertion of a PEG does not affect cerebral recovery from the stroke, it prevents the consequences of dehydration and malnutrition that may arise because of the stroke.

- Approximately one-third of patients discharged from hospital to continue tube feeding die during the first year.[32]

- Three times as many patients are discharged from hospital with a tube feed to a nursing home as are discharged home.[32]

- Most patients discharged from hospital to continue tube feeding remain dependent. A survey has shown that only 2% regained full activity, 22% undertook limited activity, 30% were housebound, 44% were bed bound and 2% were unconscious.[32]

- The presence of a PEG is a physical and psychological disability. Physical problems can be discomfort or infection at the site of insertion, leakage of feed around the tube, nausea after a feed, diarrhoea, and blocking of the tube.[34] Psychological problems include regret at loss of enjoyment of food and loss of social contact with others at mealtimes, altered body image and dependence on others.[35]

- Looking after a person with a gastrostomy at home places a considerable burden on the carer(s). In one survey, half the carers spent 15 hours or more per week visiting and caring for the patient, and some spent more than 30 hours.[34] Anxiety about care of the tube and administration of the feed is common during the early days after a patient leaves hospital. The time taken to infuse the feed, often several hours each day, limits the activities of the carer and the patient.[35] Responsibility for a patient with a severe stroke with whom communication is not possible and who needs total nursing care is both a physical and an emotional burden.[35] Carers of a stroke patient are often themselves in older age groups and have limited capacity to cope.

▌   At least 15% of patients discharged from hospital on tube feeding recover the ability to swallow, so allowing the tube to be
removed.[30] Thus it was possible to withdraw the tube in 36 (29%)
of 126 patients treated for stroke; in 19, recovery occurred more
than 6 months after it was inserted.[36] The proportion of patients
known to recover depends to some extent on the thoroughness
of re-assessment.[34,36] It is essential that reliable arrangements for
regular review, both of the patient's ability to swallow and the
social situation, are made for all patients discharged with a tube
feed to a nursing home or their own home. Such arrangements
for follow-up are complex because of the large number of health
professionals involved and a hospital protocol is needed.

5.5 Doctors' responsibilities regarding supplements, enteral tube feeds and parenteral nutrition

The doctor's role, in consultation with nursing and dietetic colleagues, is to recognise when one of these measures is indicated and
to collaborate in their implementation.

Definitions of terms related to artificial feeding and supplements
are given in Box 5.1.

Oral supplements

The provision of nourishing snacks, assistance with eating and similar
measures are the first approach to an inadequate food intake. However, such efforts may not succeed, or may be impracticable for clinical
or other reasons. Liquid or semi-solid, commercially available nutritional supplements may then have a role, to be taken in addition to, or
instead of, normal food. The effectiveness of such supplements is limited by ineffective administration to the patient or lack of patient compliance. In a careful prospective study of orthopaedic patients in the
age range 40–88 years (mean age 72), the reason for recommending a
supplement was explained to each patient by a dietitian, an explana-
tory leaflet was given, and a supplement was issued by nursing staff on
the early morning and evening drug round. Patients were given a
choice of a fruit- or milk-based supplement with a range of flavours
and were advised to sip the supplement between meals. Records of the
drinks consumed showed that patients took the supplements for only
approximately half of their hospital stay and that while the supplements were taken they took only half the volume provided. Overall,
only 14.9% of the supplements prescribed were taken but even so this
resulted in a median daily increased energy intake of 266 kcal. Thus,

Box 5.1   Definitions of terms related to artificial feeding and supplements

Medicinal supplement: In this report, the term refers to a balanced liquid or semi-solid feed prepared commercially, available in sterile portions, and authorised for prescription in the NHS by the Advisory Committee on Borderline Substances for use on medical grounds in specified disorders, including malabsorption, dysphagia and disease-related malnutrition. Liquid preparations can be used as a complete or partial source of nutrition given orally or through an enteral tube.

Nasogastric tube feed: A fine tube is introduced through the nose and pharynx so that its tip lies in the stomach. Liquid nutrients are infused through the tube either continuously using a pump or intermittently (bolus feed).

Percutaneous gastrostomy: A tube is introduced through the abdominal wall so that its tip lies in the stomach, or less commonly, in the upper small intestine. The procedure is carried out under sedation using endoscopic (PEG) or radiological control. The endoscopic technique involves passage of an endoscope through the mouth so that the entry site of the tube through the stomach wall can be visualised and its passage facilitated by pulling on a thread brought out through the mouth.

Enteral nutrition: Any technique that involves the introduction of nutrients directly into the stomach or upper small intestine through a tube.

Parenteral nutrition: The infusion of nutrients through a needle or cannula directly into a vein, so by-passing the gut. For short-term use, a peripheral vein can be used. For long-term treatment, the tip of the cannula needs to be situated in a large vein near the heart. The main dangers of the technique are blood-borne infection (septicaemia), clotting of blood around the tip of the cannula or metabolic complications.

Malabsorption: An inability of the small intestine to absorb nutrients normally.

Intestinal failure: An inability of the small intestine to absorb sufficient nutrients to maintain health.

even in this well organised mode of administration, with ample explanation and choice for patients, uptake of liquid supplements was poor, perhaps because orthopaedic patients felt little or no need for them.

Similar poor compliance was observed in a controlled trial among elderly patients, though an increased energy intake was achieved.[38] The current situation in ordinary clinical practice is revealed by a survey in 17 hospitals in the former Wessex Region. There was wide variation, but overall 14% of patients received supplements; of these 83% did not have body weight recorded and in 34% there was no documented reason why the supplements were given.[39]

From these studies it is clear that a decision to use a liquid supplement should be as part of a documented care plan for a patient who needs an extra nutritional intake of energy and/or protein, that the administration of the supplement must be well organised, and that the results should be monitored by recording the amount consumed and by regular clinical observation of nutritional state.

Nasogastric tube feeding

The advantages of an enteral tube feed are that no effort is required by the patient, swallowing difficulties may be overcome and intake is no longer dependent on appetite. A fine bore nasogastric tube through which nutrients are infused at a constant slow rate by a pump can often be tolerated by a patient for many days, weeks, or even longer. It is important to remember that this apparently simple procedure is regarded in law as a medical treatment and the permission of a competent patient is required after adequate explanation (see section 2.6). A clear indication for a nasogastric tube feed is a patient with a normally functioning intestine who, for more than a few days, cannot eat or drink. A relative indication is for treatment of a patient who, despite efforts to increase oral intake, does not take enough nutrients to sustain health or restore lost tissue through apathy, weakness, anorexia or unwillingness. A tube feed can also be used as a supplement to normal food, often as an infusion over night, so that intestinal absorption is continuous throughout 24 hours. This may be necessary when there has been very severe weight loss and the patient will benefit from a nutrient intake greater than can be achieved by mouth, or when intestinal absorption is greatly impaired, for example after major resection of the small bowel.

Nutrition or hydration via a nasogastric (or gastrostomy) tube does not necessarily avoid pulmonary aspiration. Pulmonary aspiration may be due to aspiration of secretions from the mouth and nose or reflux of gastric contents up to the pharynx. The latter may be minimised when considered necessary by placing the tip of an infusion tube near the duodeno–jejunal junction using an endoscope.

Percutaneous endoscopic gastrostomy (PEG)

If nasogastric intubation is likely to be needed for several weeks or longer, especially if it is poorly tolerated, percutaneous gastrostomy can be performed using an endoscopic or radiological technique. If the procedure is performed in very ill patients there is risk of early death. The Confidential Enquiry into Perioperative Deaths has recorded 12 deaths within three days of endoscopic placement, and a total of 17 deaths within 30 days, and recommended that the procedure should not be performed unless the patient has a reasonable likelihood of survival beyond this period.[33] There is a small complication rate of

CASE STUDY 5 – Mrs B, aged 65, was admitted to hospital with acute abdominal pain and vomiting. On examination she was overnourished and had a BMI of 28. Investigations showed that she had small bowel obstruction. This failed to respond to conservative therapy and three days later adhesions were divided at laparotomy. On the sixth postoperative day a further episode of intestinal obstruction was followed by signs of peritonism. At a second laparotomy a 40-cm segment of gangrenous small intestine was resected. On the fifth day, following her second laparotomy, partial wound dehiscence occurred and the following day an enterocutaneous fistula developed. Mrs B was pyrexial, apathetic and depressed. Investigation showed that the fistula originated from the site of the anastomosis and there was no proximal small bowel dilatation. After consultation between the nutritional support and surgical teams, it was decided to provide enteral nutrition via a fine bore nasogastric feeding tube. The fistula closed after three weeks and the wound healed after a further two weeks of enteral feeding. A normal diet was then started and the patient was subsequently discharged from hospital well.

Comment – Overnutrition does not preclude the subsequent development of undernutrition and, by the time the wound dehiscence and entero-cutaneous fistula developed, this patient had received no oral nutrition for 16 days. Her lack of nutritional intake, with the metabolic response to surgical injury and sepsis, led to a serum albumin of 24 g/l, marked loss of lean body mass, a weight loss of 9 kg, apathy and depression. The joint decision of the multidisciplinary nutritional support and surgical team to give enteral nutrition was justified by subsequent events. Parenteral nutrition is not always needed in the treatment of an enterocutaneous fistula, provided that the fluid losses are not too large and there is no other contra-indication to use of the enteral route.

insertion in any patient due to sedation or intra-abdominal hazards such as pneumo-peritoneum, haemorrhage or peritonitis. The commonest long-term sequelae are pulmonary aspiration or infection at the site of introduction, which occurred, for example, in 18% and 17% respectively of 126 patients with stroke in one series followed for a mean of 31 months.[36]

Since introduction of a gastrostomy tube is a long-term measure with major consequences for the patient and carers, proper consultation is indicated before it is inserted. Once begun, gastrostomy feeding is difficult to stop and a clear goal should, if possible, be established at the outset. One aim may be to allow time for possible recovery of swallowing. Alternatively, the tube can be inserted to maintain adequate nutrition throughout the remainder of a patient's life in cases where the ability to swallow will never be regained.

It is important that patients and carers are not under any misapprehension about the purpose and limitations of the treatment. For example, in motor neurone disease maintenance of nutrition avoids any component of muscle weakness due to undernutrition but it does not delay the progression of neurological deterioration. It is possible that the patient might wish to discontinue tube feeding in the last stages of the disease, if the discomfort of treatment outweighs the benefit.

Failure to achieve a goal, as in long-standing coma or persistent vegetative state, may lead to a decision that the treatment is futile and withdrawal should be considered, following accepted procedures.[40]

Parenteral nutrition

Parenteral nutrition is reserved for patients with intestinal failure, defined as an inability of the gut to absorb adequate nutrients to maintain health. This situation may be temporary, as during prolonged ileus, or long-term, as after resection of the majority of the small intestine or because of disease of the small intestine such as pseudo-obstruction. Parenteral nutrition requires meticulous organisation if dangerous complications, such as septicaemia, are to be avoided. It is an expensive though potentially life-saving measure when used correctly in appropriate circumstances. Details of the technique are outside the scope of this report but the development of a specialist nutrition support team in every acute hospital to organise and supervise its use (see below) is a desirable policy that yields both clinical efficiency and economic savings.[41]

5.6 Doctors as members of hospital nutrition support teams

In many hospitals, a nutrition support team advises on, or undertakes, all artificial feeding. Through experience gained and the use of protocols, such a team can greatly improve the results of artificial feeding, diminish complications and reduce costs through standardisation of indications and supplies.[41]

A nutrition support team is usually composed of a doctor, a nurse, a dietitian and a pharmacist.[5] The team typically assumes responsibility for the nutritional care of patients with complicated nutritional problems who require a tube feed or parenteral nutrition. The team also trains patients, and/or their carers, in the relevant technique when they are ready to leave hospital but still need artificial nutrition.

As a member of the team, a doctor advises on clinical issues, may insert central intravenous feeding lines and, in approximately two-thirds of existing teams, acts as leader.[5] Appropriate training of the doctor for this specialist role is desirable.

Doctors employed in hospital who have special clinical responsibility for nutritional care have responsibilities at the interface between primary and secondary care. They liaise with GPs when patients with a nutritional problem, especially those who continue artificial nutrition, leave hospital, and also need to be available for advice when a difficult nutritional problem arises in primary care. The job description of such a hospital doctor should reflect this commitment to give help in the community.

5.7 A doctor's contribution to nutritional policy for a hospital trust

As stated in Chapter 6, advantages would follow if hospital catering were to be regarded as a clinical aspect of management rather than as a 'hotel service'. Trusts are encouraged to establish a nutrition steering or co-ordinating group. Such a body should have the same status as existing drug and therapeutics committees. Nutrition steering groups are being established by some hospital trusts with representation from management, the catering department, dietetics, nursing, medicine and the pharmacy (see also Chapter 7). A doctor with a special interest and experience in nutrition has an important role in contributing to development of nutritional policy in this way.

References

1 Baker JP, Detsky AS, Wesson DE *et al.* Nutritional assessment: a comparison of clinical judgement and objective measurements. *N Eng J Med* 1982; **306**: 969–72.

2 Jeejeebhoy KN, Baker JP, Wolman SL *et al.* Critical evaluation of the role of clinical assessment and body composition studies in patients with malnutrition and after total parenteral nutrition. *Am J Clin Nutr* 1982; **35**: 1117–27.

3 Windsor JA, Hill GL. Weight loss with physiological impairment: a basic indicator of surgical risk. *Ann Surg* 1988; **207**: 290–96.

4 Audit Commission. *Acute hospital portfolio: Catering, review of national findings.* Wetherby: Audit Commission Publications, 2001.

5 British Artificial Nutrition Survey (BANS). *Trends in artificial nutrition in the U.K. during 1996-2000.* Maidenhead: British Association For Parenteral and Artificial Nutrition (BAPEN), 2001

6 Department of Health. *Report on health and social subjects, 41. Dietary reference values for food energy and nutrients for the United Kingdom: a report of the panel on dietary values of the Committee on Medical Aspects of Food Policy.* London: HMSO, 1991.

7 Department of Health. *Nutrition guidelines for hospital catering.* Prepared by the Hospital Catering Project Team of the Health of the Nation Nutrition Task Force.Wetherby: DH, 1995.

8 Allison, SP (ed). *Hospital food as treatment.* Maidenhead: British Association for Parenteral and Enteral Nutrition, 1999.

9 Barton, AD, Beigg, CL, Macdonald, IA, Allison, SP. High food wastage and low nutritional intakes in hospital patients. *Clin Nutr* 2000; **19**: 445–9.

10 Edwards J, Nash A. Measuring the wasteline. *Health Services Journal*, November: 26–27.

11 Todd EA, Hunt P, Crowe PJ, Royle GT. What do patients eat in hospital? *Hum Nutr Appl Nutr* 1984; **38A**: 294–7.

12 McWirter JP, Pennington CR. Incidence and recognition of malnutrition in hospital. *BMJ* 1994: **308**: 945–8.

13 Corish CA, Kennedy NP. Protein-energy undernutrition in hospital in-patients: review article. *Br J Nutr* 2000; **83**: 575–91.

14 Akner G, Cederholm, T. Treatment of protein-energy malnutrition in chronic nonmalignant disorders. *Am J Clin Nutr* 2001; **74**: 6–24.

15 Tucker H. Cost containment through nutrition intervention. *Nutrition Reviews* 1996; **54**: 111–21.

16 Lewis SJ, Egger M, Sylvester A, Thomas S. Early enteral feeding versus 'nil by mouth' after gastrointestinal surgery: systematic review and meta-analysis of controlled trials. *BMJ* 2001; **323**: 773–6.

17 Finch S, Doyle W, Lowe C *et al. National Diet and Nutrition Survey: people aged 65 years and over. Volume 1: Report of the diet and nutrition survey*. London: The Stationery Office, 1998.

18 Elia M, Stratton RJ. How much undernutrition is there in hospitals? *Br J Nutr* 2000; **84**: 257–9.

19 Corish CA, Flood P, Mulligan S, Kennedy NP. Apparent low frequency of undernutrition in Dublin hospital in-patients: should we review the anthropometric thresholds for clinical practice? *Br J Nutr* 2000; **84**; 325–35.

20 Bastow MD, Rawlings J, Allison SP. Undernutrition, hypothermia, and injury in elderly women with fractured femur: an injury response to altered metabolism? *Lancet* 1983; **i**: 143–6.

21 Bastow MD, Rawlings J, Allison SP. Benefits of supplementary tube feeding after fractured neck of femur: a randomised controlled trial. *BMJ* 1983; **287**: 1589–92.

22 Thomas AJ, Bunker V, Hinks LJ *et al.* Energy, protein, zinc and copper status of twenty-one elderly inpatients: analysed dietary intake and biochemical indices. *Br J Nutr* 1988; **59**: 181–91.

23 Olin AO, Osterberg P, Hadell K *et al.* Energy-enriched hospital food to improve energy intake in elderly patients. *J Parent Ent Nutr* 1996; **20**: 93–7.

24 Gall MJ, Grimble GK, Reeve NJ, Thomas SJ. Effect of providing fortified meals and between-meal snacks on energy and protein intake of hospital patients. *Clin Nutr* 1998; **17**: 259–64.

25 Barton AD, Beigg CI, Macdonald IA, Allison SP. A recipe for improving food intakes in elderly hospitalized patients. *Clin Nutr* 2000; **19**: 451–4.

26 McWhirter JP, Pennington CR. A comparison between oral and nasogastric nutritional supplements in malnourished patients. *Nutrition* 1996; **12**: 502–6.

27 Ardron ME, Main AN. Management of constipation. *BMJ* 1990; **300**: 1400.

28 Evans E, Stock AL. Dietary intake of geriatric patients in hospital. *Nutr Metabol* 1971; **13**: 21–35.

29 Gariballa SE. Nutritional factors in stroke. *Br J Nutr* 2000; **84**: 5–17.

30 Gariballa SE, Taub N, Parker SG, Castleden CM. A randomised controlled trial of oral nutritional supplements following acute stroke. *JPEN* 1998; **22**: 315–19.

31 Barer DH. The natural history and functional consequences of dysphagia after hemispheric stroke. *J Neurol Psych* 1989; **52**: 236–41.

32 Elia M, Stratton RJ, Holden C *et al.* Home enteral tube feeding following cerebrovascular accident. *Clin Nutr* 2001; **20**: 27–30.

33 Rosin RD, Hoile R. Percutaneous endoscopic gastrostomy (PEG). *Report of the National Confidential Enquiry into Perioperative Deaths 1996/7*. London: DH, National Confidential Enquiry into Perioperative Deaths, 1998: 43–45.

34 Verhoef MJ, Van Rosendaal GM. Patient outcomes related to percutaneous endoscopic gastrostomy placement. *J Clin Gastroenterol* 2001; **32**: 49–53.

35 Rickman J. Percutaneous endoscopic gastrostomy: psychological effects. *Br J Nurs* 1998; **7**: 723–9.

36 James A, Kapur K, Hawthorne AB. Long-term outcome of percutaneous endoscopic gastrostomy feeding in patients with dysphagic stroke. *Age Ageing* 1998; **27**: 671–6.

37 Lawson RM, Doshi MK, Ingoe LE *et al*. Compliance of orthopaedic patients with postoperative oral nutritional supplementation. *Clin Nutr* 2000: **19**: 171–5.

38 Hogarth MB, Marshall P, Lovat LB *et al*. Nutritional supplementation in elderly medical in-patients: a double-blind placebo-controlled trial. *Age Ageing* 1996: **25**: 453–7.

39 Brosnan S, Margetts B, Munro J *et al*. on behalf of the Wessex Dietetic Managers Group. The reported use of dietary supplements (sip feeds) in hospitals in Wessex, UK. *Clin Nutr* 2001: **20**: 445–9.

40 British Medical Association. *Withholding and withdrawing life prolonging medical treatment: guidance for decision making.* London: British Medical Association, 1999.

41 Lennard-Jones JE (ed). *A positive approach to nutrition as treatment.* London: King's Fund Centre, 1992.

6 | Provision of food in hospital

SUMMARY

▮ Doctors should be aware of their patients' nutritional intake during their stay in hospital.

▮ Doctors should make themselves familiar with the aspects of food service pertinent to their patients.

▮ Doctors must ensure that any act or omission on their part does not compromise patients' nutrition.

6.1 Introduction

Hospitals are viewed as institutions and institutional catering has a poor reputation.[1] Even before patients have sampled the food, they are often prepared to dislike it, and when compared with other eating settings, hospitals receive the lowest ratings.[2] This phenomenon is often referred to as 'institutional stereotyping' and is caused, in part, by poor variety and presentation of the food and a poor physical dining setting. It is important, therefore, that doctors appreciate that the provision of an adequate and balanced diet forms an integral part of a patient's treatment and involves more than just the delivery of a meal to a patient. An understanding of the food service process will ensure the integration of food into the overall treatment. A number of previous studies[3,4] have identified the critical areas. This chapter highlights the important aspects of food service for patients.

6.2 Better hospital food: the NHS Plan

The NHS Plan, *A plan for investment, a plan for reform,*[5] sets out targets for the improvement of hospital food in England (Scotland, Wales and Northern Ireland will be developing similar measures in due course). The Better Hospital Food Project was launched in May 2001 to implement these improvements and is supported by information on the website, www.betterhospitalfood.com

Six essential targets were scheduled for implementation by December 2001. These were to:

▮ Implement the new menu framework. This describes the meals to be provided and the minimum amount of choice to be offered.

▪ Make food available to patients throughout the 24-hour period. This is to be achieved through better provision of food in the ward kitchen, 'snack boxes' and 'lite bites' (micowavable meals for one).

▪ Offer each day three of the dishes developed especially for the NHS by a panel of leading chefs.

▪ Promote the food services in each trust by means of the NHS menu brochure to be offered to each patient.

▪ Provide snacks with the mid-afternoon and evening beverages.

▪ Provide the nutritional requirements for a variety of patient needs; this should be checked by a state-registered dietitian.

The implementation of this project is managed by NHS Estates and will be part of the performance assessment framework for hospital trusts in England. The NHS Plan for England is a 10-year plan, and it is anticipated that food service developments in the NHS will continue. The Better Hospital Food Project is a four-year plan backed up by £40 million of investment funding.

6.3 The menu

The printed menu is the primary means of communicating what food is on offer, and generally the first opportunity patients have to see what is available. Food is selected by name, not by sensory or other evaluation, and patients may be reluctant to eat in hospital because dishes are imprecisely described, so they may be unsure of exactly what to expect.[6] Meal selection needs to be made from a menu which clearly communicates what is available, is in the appropriate language, is unambiguous, is easily read and understood, and does not give the impression of being 'institutional'. The Better Hospital Food initiative in England requires trusts to provide a high quality brochure for each patient describing the food service. Menu choice and variety are important, particularly when patients have been in hospital for any length of time; choice should also reflect and be appropriate to patients' medical and other needs. A variety of dishes, flavours, colours and textures can help.[7]

6.4 Ordering

Where meals are ordered in advance, it is important that menu cards are accurately completed. Advice and assistance in completing menu cards should be available; various portion sizes should be offered and provided; and menu cards should be checked by ward staff for accuracy and completeness before being sent to the kitchen. New patients should be given the opportunity to order their own food. Consideration should therefore be given to a system whereby patients are able to make their meal choice at the point and time of consumption.

Treatments and procedures requiring a period of nil by mouth beforehand reduce food intake, sometimes beyond the necessary fasting period. A patient may have had nothing to eat all morning only to have the treatment delayed or postponed to a later date.[8] Patients may need to fast for only 4-6 hours preoperatively, but in practice this is rarely adhered to.[9] Care should be taken to ensure that if patients are nil by mouth and their procedure is postponed, provision is made for them to have something to eat. The re-development of the ward kitchen and the NHS 'snack box' is designed to meet this need.

6.5 Food regeneration

Where regeneration occurs at ward level, meals need to be heated for approximately 45-60 minutes. Hot meals, therefore, cannot be produced on demand. Similarly, once food has been reheated, it can be held at the appropriate temperature only for a short time before the quality begins to deteriorate. For food safety reasons, it must not be cooled down for reheating later on.

6.6 Service

The attitude of staff who serve and deliver meals can affect patients' satisfaction and perception of the quality of a meal.[10,11] Adverse comments about the food made by individual members of staff can affect not only consumers' views of the food but also the amount actually consumed.[12] All staff, including medical and nursing staff, should be aware of this.

6.7 The meal

The 'patient meal' comprises not only the food but also the patient and the situation in which consumption takes place.

The food

Temperature Temperatures affect many aspects of the food and, in combination with its sensory properties, often determines how well it is liked.[13] When food is served at unfamiliar temperatures, enjoyment can be affected and it may be rejected because it is not considered appropriate. When served at the 'correct' temperature, enjoyment and acceptability are at their highest.[14] Serving food at the correct temperature, whether it is 'hot' or 'cold', is therefore essential to the enjoyment of meals.

Portion size For many elderly patients, the sight of a large meal is overwhelming and may deter them from eating. Patients should be given the opportunity to select portion sizes appropriate to their appetite.

The patient

Nature of the illness All staff need to be sensitive to the nature of the patient's underlying illness. The aim must be to ensure that food is appropriate and is eaten. Advice should be sought and taken from dietitians and food service managers.

Eating 'disabilities' Food is of value only when consumed and the ability of patients to feed themselves can be impaired by a variety of factors. Adequate help by nursing staff, domestic assistance, or relatives should be available to patients where required.

Appetite Many conditions requiring hospital admission lead to a diminished appetite. Drug treatment, unfamiliar surroundings, anaesthetics and anxiety may compound this problem. In order to develop an effective treatment plan, doctors need to be aware of what the patient is eating and the effects various treatments have on appetite.

The situation

Mealtimes Mealtimes (along with visiting) are often the highlight of the patient's day, frequently being the only break from the monotony and routine of their stay in hospital.[15,16] Meals should not, therefore, be undermined by other ward routines. The timing of meals is important and patients may feel more relaxed and at ease in the unnatural surroundings when timing of mealtimes is as close as possible to those at home.[17] One common comment is that patients would prefer meals, particularly in the evening, to be served later. The amount of food consumed can be predicted by the subjective state of hunger, prior stomach content – particularly the amount of protein – and the length of time since food was last eaten. Individually these factors are small but collectively may account for 28% of the variation.[18] The appropriate 'spacing' and timings of meals is, therefore, important. The Better Hospital Food Project addresses these issues of mealtimes, the 24-hour availability of food and increased opportunity to eat during the patient's day.

Social importance of meals Meals and mealtimes should be an enjoyable experience, and patient satisfaction and perception of the food service and meals are closely interwoven with social, physical and emotional aspects of the environment.[11] These social factors are equally, if not more, important in determining which food is chosen and how much is eaten.[19]

Eating is usually considered a social activity and, in general, more food is consumed in company than in isolation.[20] This 'social facilitation' applies to a variety of eating situations, and preliminary results suggest that it holds true for hospital wards, where more food is consumed in the company of others.[21] The presence of nursing staff during mealtimes has been suggested as a way of benefiting the nutritional (and nursing) care of patients.[22] The Essence of Care: Patient-Focussed Benchmarking Project specifically focuses on setting standards for staff availability at mealtimes.[23]

Length of wait Making people wait for meals affects both their opinion of the service[24] and the liking for the food consumed.[25] Meals need to be served on time and not delayed for domestic ward routines.

6.8 Feedback

Many of the failings in the food service system, and much of the food wasted at ward level, can be attributed to weak (or lack of) feedback and communication between the ward and the hospital food service department. It often means that patients' needs – for example, nil by mouth – are not communicated and that too much food is ordered, to ensure that it does not run out.

Hospital food service systems are very information-intensive but the requirement is often overlooked when systems are planned and installed. Adequate provision for information and feedback needs to be considered in any new build or update. Food consumption, along with other medical procedures, should be monitored at ward level, and appropriate follow-up action taken to ensure that meals are integrated into part of the overall treatment and not considered as just a minor 'refuelling' process.

6.9 Conclusions

Adequate nutrition is an integral and important part of patients' treatment, with the most cost-effective solution being the provision of an adequate and balanced diet provided from hospital food. However, if it is to be of nutritional value, food must be consumed; when it has been prepared but not consumed scarce resources are wasted.

The nutritional status of patients is the responsibility of all staff, doctors included, who need to ensure that food reaches patients in optimum condition, at the correct time and temperature, and that it is actually consumed. This should not be subsumed by medical and other ward procedures. Only then can food become part of the treatment.

References

1   Bender AE. Institutional malnutrition. *BMJ* 1984; **288**: 92–3.
2   Cardello AV. The role of image, stereotypes, and expectations on the acceptance and consumption of rations. In Marriott BM (ed) *Not eating enough*. Washington: National Academy Press, 1995
3   Allison SP (ed). *Hospital food as treatment. A report by a working party of the British Association for Parenteral and Enteral Nutrition*. Maidenhead: BAPEN, 1999.
4   Edwards JSA, Edwards A and Salmon JA. Food service management in hospitals. *Int J Contemporary Hospitality Management* 2000; **12**(4): 262–6.
5   Department of Health. *A plan for investment, a plan for reform*. London: DH, 2000.
6   Fenton J, Eves A, Kipps M, O'Donnell CD. The Nutritional Implications of Foodservice practices and food acceptability on the diets of elderly patients in continuing care. *Hygiene and Nutrition in Foodservice and Catering* 1997; **1**: 281–98.
7   Rolls BJ. Sensory-specific satiety and variety in the meal. In Meiselman HL (ed) *Dimensions of the meal*. Gaithersburg, Maryland: Aspen Publishers Inc, 2000: 107–16.
8   Schenker S. Malnutrition in hospital. *British Nutrition Foundation Bulletin* 1993; **23**: 131–6.
9   Hung P. Preoperative fasting of patients undergoing elective surgery. *B J Nurs* 1992; **1**(6): 286–7.
10   Gregoire MB. Quality of patient meal service in hospitals: delivery of meals by dietary employees vs delivery by nursing employees. *J Am Diet Assoc* 1994; **10**: 1129–34.
11   Dubé L, Trudean E, Bélanger M-C. Determining the complexity of patient satisfaction with foodservices. *J Am Diet Assoc* 1994; **4**: 394–401.
12   Cardello AV, Bell R, Kramer FM. Attitudes of consumers toward military and other institutional food. *Food Quality and Preference* 1996; **1**: 7–20.
13   Zellner DA, Stewart WF, Rozin P, Brown JM. Effect of temperature and expectations on liking for beverages. *Physiol Behav* 1988; **44**(1): 61–8.
14   Cardello AV, Maller O. Acceptability of water, selected beverages and foods as a function of serving temperature. *J Food Sci* 1982; **47**: 1549–52.
15   Glew G. Food preferences of hospital patients. *Proc Nutr Soc* 1970; **29**(2): 339–43.
16   Association of Community Health Councils of England and Wales. *Hungry in*

hospital? London: Association of Community Health Councils of England and Wales, 1997.

17   McGlone PC, Dickerson JWT and Davies GJ. The feeding of patients in hospital: a review. *J Roy Soc Health* 1995; **23**: 282–8.

18   de Castro JM. Physiological, environmental and subjective determinants on food intake in humans: a meal pattern analysis. *Physiol Behav* 1988; **44**: 651–9.

19   Bell R, Meiselman HL. The role of eating environments in determining food choice, In: Marshall DW (ed) *Food choice and the consumer.* Texas: Culinary and Hospitality Industry Publications, 1995; 292–310.

20   de Castro JM and de Castro ES. Spontaneous meal patterns of humans: influence of the presence of other people. *Am J Clin Nutr* 1989; **50**: 237–47.

21   Hartwell HH, Edwards JSA. *Comparison of mean energy intake between eating situations in a NHS hospital – a pilot study.* Poster at the Annual Meeting of the British Association for Parenteral and Enteral Nutrition. Harrogate, 28-30 November, 2000.

22   Wykes R. The nutritional and nursing benefits of social mealtimes, *Nursing Times* 1997; **93**(4): 32–4.

23   Department of Health. *The essence of care: patient-focussed benchmarking for health care practitioners.* London: Department of Health, 2001.

24   Meiselman HL. Determining consumer preference in institutional food service. In: Livingston GE (ed) *Food service systems analysis, design and planning.* London: Academic Press, 1979: 127–53.

25   Edwards JSA. The effects of queuing on food preferences. *Int J Hospitality Management* 1984; **3**(2): 83–5.

PART FOUR

Clinical governance, education and training

7 | The recognition of nutrition in clinical governance

SUMMARY

- Doctors should recognise that proper nutritional care is fundamental to good clinical practice.

- It is the doctor's responsibility to ensure that information concerning nutritional status and care is properly documented in the patient's clinical record, that appropriate action has been taken to deal with any nutritional problem, and that the patient and/or carer are kept fully informed.

- Doctors should ensure that adequate details of their patients' nutritional status and care, including psychosocial aspects, are communicated effectively to relevant clinical colleagues. This is particularly important at the time of admission to and discharge from hospital.

- Doctors should ensure that they receive appropriate training and updates on nutritional care as part of their lifelong learning.

- Doctors should join with colleagues from other disciplines in developing local nutritional care practice, policies, standards and audits based on national guidelines.

7.1 Introduction

Clinical governance is about assuring quality of care – making sure that patients are well treated in every respect. It means seeing each health care experience through the eyes of the patient, and making changes to improve the way things are done. In this chapter, issues identified in the previous chapters are examined in the context of clinical governance. Doctors are central to clinical governance. Working closely with other health professionals and managers, they are well placed to help ensure good practice.[1]

7.2 Clinical governance and nutritional care

The report has considered the evidence for regarding nutritional screening and assessment, the provision of hospital food, feeding practices, and artificial nutrition when necessary, as essential elements of nutritional care. It has drawn attention to the related medico-legal and ethical issues. The management of under- and overnutrition in primary care and among older people in residential and nursing homes has also been examined. Nutritional care, in whatever setting, should be fully integrated into clinical programmes and developed within a framework of clinical governance.

There are several aspects of nutritional care that make it well suited to a clinical governance approach:

▪ Nutrition is clearly linked to health, well-being and clinical recovery.

▪ The quality of food and nutrition are high on the list of patient and carer concerns.

▪ There are simple measuring tools for assessing nutritional status and monitoring consumption.

▪ Making improvements can save resources in the longer term.

▪ A wide range of staff are involved in preparing and providing food.

▪ Many of the lessons learned can be generalised into other areas of care.

7.3 Setting standards

Undernutrition

Many hospitals have developed their own clinical guidelines and standards based on national recommendations that have appeared over recent years. With particular regard to undernutrition, the Nuffield Trust report, *Managing nutrition in hospital: a recipe for quality,*[2] calls for clear national standards – perhaps through appropriate national service frameworks and/or the National Institute for Clinical Excellence (NICE) – for the following aspects of nutritional care:

▪ nutritional quality and palatability of hospital food
▪ preparation, distribution and serving of meals
▪ nutritional screening, assessment and monitoring
▪ feeding practices
▪ referral protocols
▪ nutritional support protocols
▪ audit protocols
▪ education and training.

Progress towards national standards has been made in all these areas. For hospital catering, for example, the NHS Plan[3] outlines targets to be achieved in improving the quality and availability of food to patients. Standards for nutritional screening, assessment, and monitoring in the community have been proposed in widely accepted guidelines recently published by the Malnutrition Advisory Group of the British Association for Parenteral and Enteral Nutrition (BAPEN).[4] Feeding practices have been the subject of a recent national 'benchmarking' exercise.[5]

In primary care, there is less clear guidance about undernutrition in terms of national standards. For one key client group, the *National Service Framework for Older People* puts forward some general objectives.[6] These include the introduction of a single assessment process in health and social care to ensure that older people's needs are assessed and evaluated fully. Where older people are likely to receive intensive forms of support, including permanent admission to a care home, intermediate care or intensive support at home, professionals should undertake a comprehensive old age assessment. In doing this, they should include an assessment of needs with regard to eating and drinking. For the wider population, the main standard concerned with nutritional imbalance focuses on increasing the consumption of fruit and vegetables, outlined in the *National cancer plan*[7] and endorsed in the NHS Plan.

Overnutrition

With regard to overnutrition, standards are centred around obesity and excessive intake of fatty foods. For England these are set down in the *National Service Framework for Coronary Heart Disease.*[8] All NHS trusts and other health bodies should have agreed policies on the promotion of healthy eating and the prevention and control of obesity among patients and the wider public.

The main clinical setting for these interventions is in primary care, with referral to secondary specialist nutritional and dietetic care for cases at highest risk. Primary care teams are required to have developed and maintained a register of patients with existing heart disease in order to prioritise them for advice and treatment aimed at secondary prevention, including dietary advice for those with hypercholesterolaemia or obesity. A second phase adds high risk patients who have not yet developed heart disease. Protocols for these interventions should be agreed locally and should take on board both the appropriate training of primary care staff in providing nutrition and dietary advice, and minimum standards with regard to community dietetic support. Further impetus to these developments is provided by the National Service Framework (NSF) for people with diabetes.[9]

7.4 Practical aspects at the clinical level

Nutritional care is fundamental to good clinical practice, and it is recommended that every doctor should help improve the quality of nutritional care by contributing, together with other relevant staff, to a comprehensive clinical governance approach. For example, the doctor should ensure that standards are maintained in respect of:

▮   *Record-keeping:* key information concerning nutritional status and care is documented in the patient's clinical record.

▮   *Clinical management:* appropriate action based on sound evidence is taken in order to investigate and deal with any nutritional problem.

▮   *Communication with the patient/carer:* timely information is given to the patient and/or carer, and their questions are answered openly and honestly.

▮   *Communication with clinical colleagues:* adequate details of their patients' nutritional status and care, and relevant psychosocial status, are communicated effectively to relevant clinical colleagues. This is particularly important on admission and discharge.

▮   *Lifelong learning:* doctors should ensure that they receive appropriate further training and updates on nutritional matters as part of lifelong learning.

▮   *Development of a clinical governance framework.*

7.5 Clinical 'benchmarking'

Doctors should join with colleagues from other disciplines in developing an approach to the clinical governance of nutritional care. One such initiative developed at national level is clinical 'benchmarking'. This is a structured way of looking at shortfalls in the nutritional care pathway, expounded in *The essence of care – a national nursing initiative.*[5] 'Food and Nutrition' is one of eight benchmark areas aimed at ensuring that patients are screened on admission, and that appropriate action is taken according to nutritional needs. It considers such aspects as: policies, procedures and guidelines; staffing issues; education and training; information and communication; facilities and equipment; patient-specific needs; teamwork issues. Through a shared approach, it allows direct comparisons between wards in order to arrive at an agreed action plan.

7.6 Nutritional care at trust level

Management arrangements for co-ordinating nutritional care at trust level will vary from trust to trust, but would be expected to involve a multidisciplinary co-ordinating committee (eg a nutrition steering group), led a by a senior nurse, doctor or allied health professional (see Example of good practice below). Trusts must encourage doctors to identify a lead clinician responsible for championing nutrition and nutritional care across all disciplines within the trust. Developing clinical governance for nutritional care would be expected to form part of the remit of this committee, but responsibility for ensuring that a suitable approach is taken should be borne by the trust clinical governance lead.

EXAMPLE OF GOOD PRACTICE – St George's Hospital, London

The hospital has established a Nutrition Strategy Committee, led by a consultant physican.

The terms of reference are:

- To bring together the managers and professionals involved in the provision of 'normal' food and nutritional support within the trust.
- To advise... the medical director and chief executive on matters relevant to nutritional practice and policy.
- To manage a nutrition support team (NST) and co-ordinate nutritional support throughout the trust.
- To produce guidelines for the universal nutritional assessment of hospital patients, for appropriate nutritional management and referral to the NST.
- To advise on the purchase of suitable products relevant to dietetic therapy and nutritional support.
- To develop a strategy for improving the nutritional education of health professionals.
- To agree clinical standards for structure, process and outcome in the provision of nutritional care, which may then be applied to audit and the contracting process.
- To liaise with individual specialties through the existing service delivery unit structure. Where necessary, to co-opt additional members [on to the Committee]
- To review expenditure on catering and nutritional support in order to improve cost-effectiveness and quality.

Membership of the Committee comprises:

- manager, dietetic services
- pharmaceutical manager
- director of nursing
- estates director
- director of quality
- business manager
- Faculty of Healthcare Sciences representative
- health promotion hospital co-ordinator
- consultant clinician.

In primary care, similar arrangements should be set up under the auspices of primary care trusts (or their equivalent). These could oversee and co-ordinate the nutritional elements of national service frameworks (such as coronary heart disease (CHD), health of older people, diabetes), NICE guidance, the NHS Plan, and other relevant national or local priorities.

Box 7.1 outlines some recommendations for addressing nutrition within a clinical governance framework in NHS trusts and strategic health authorities.*

7.7 Performance assessment

Clinical governance should concentrate on what matters to patients, particularly in terms of the following domains of the National Performance Assessment Framework (NPAF):

- *fair access* (eg to nutritious and acceptable food and help with feeding for vulnerable people from diverse social and cultural groups, care groups etc)
- *effective delivery of appropriate care* (eg nutritional assessment, referral for nutritional support, supplements etc)
- *patient/carer experience* (eg perceptions of quality of nutritional care, including food provision and feeding support)
- *health outcomes* (eg impact of nutritional care on such indicators as changes in level of nutritional risk, post-operative complications, case fatality etc).

The two other NPAF domains should also be monitored:

- *efficiency* (eg lengths of stay, prescribing of nutritional supplements, catering costs, etc)
- *health improvement* (eg readmission rates, consultation rates, mortality rates).

This is a sizeable list and audits will need to be prioritised. Detailed guidance on performance assessment at local level with regard to obesity prevention and control has been provided by the Faculty of Public Health Medicine.[10]

7.8 Resource implications

Clinical governance is not resource-neutral. Audits, bench-marking, sharing learning and implementing improvements all cost money. For this work to go forward effectively, nutritional care must be accepted

---

*For further information on clinical governance, contact the NHS Clinical Governance Support Team, 2nd Floor, 6 Millstone Lane, Leicester, LE1 5ZW. Email: support@ncgstnhs.uk

Box 7.1 Nutritional clinical governance: recommendations to NHS trusts and strategic health authorities

For the trust:

- The important role of nutritional care in the delivery of the NHS Plan and national service frameworks (eg CHD, older people's health and diabetes) should be recognised.

- For nutrition to have the status it deserves within trusts, the board should nominate a member as 'nutrition champion' and state its commitment to including nutritional care within the overall clinical governance framework.

- Each trust should establish a multiprofessional nutritional advisory group (or equivalent) with sufficient powers to oversee, co-ordinate and integrate agreed nutritional policies and practices into everyday patient care.

- Everyone – from kitchen staff to consultants – should have a clear understanding of roles and responsibilities in the provision of food, feeding and nutritional care.

- Nutritional care should be included in the trust's strategy and structure for clinical governance and audit.

- The trust should provide sufficient resources for proper clinical governance of nutritional care.

- The trust should be able to respond positively to sound cases made by clinical teams for service changes arising from a clinical governance approach.

- Patient advocacy and liaison services should be fully involved in the above arrangements.

For primary care organisations and strategic health authorities/boards:

- Clinical governance of nutritional care should be incorporated into service level agreements (or equivalent) with trusts and primary care practices.

- Standards should include an appropriate level of dietetic support for primary care, particularly with regard to undernutrition, diabetes, obesity and hyperlipidaemia.

- Nutritional care must comprise a key element of the performance assessment of trusts and primary care, and be conducted in sufficient depth and detail to learn useful practical lessons.

- Health authorities/boards have a role in sharing good practice with regard to nutritional care.

as a priority and appropriate resources must be made available. Funding can usually be garnered from audit, quality and IT budgets. Within trusts, clear commitment at board level is required, and a duty should be placed on the trust clinical governance lead to ensure that sufficient resources are brought to bear. Patient advocacy and liaison services can also play a part in this. Contract negotiations with health care commissioners should reflect the requirement for adequate funding of clinical governance.

References

1 NHS Executive. *A first class service: consultation document on quality in the new NHS.* London: DH, 1998, HSC1998/113.

2 Maryon Davis A, Bristow A. *Managing nutrition in hospital: a recipe for quality.* Monograph No. 8. London: The Nuffield Trust, 1999.

3 Department of Health. *The NHS Plan. A plan for investment, a plan for reform.* London: DH, 2000, Cm 4818–1.

4 Elia M (ed). *MAG guidelines for detection and management of malnutrition.* London: MAG/BAPEN, 2001.

5 Department of Health. *Essence of care: Patient-focused benchmarking for health care practitioners.* London: DH, 2001.

6 Department of Health. *National Service Framework for Older People.* London: DH, 2001.

7 Department of Health. *The NHS cancer plan.* London: DH, 2001.

8 Department of Health. *National Service Framework for Coronary Heart Disease.* London: DH, 2000.

9 Department of Health. *National Service Framework for Diabetes.* London: DH, 2002.

10 Department of Health. *The essence of care: a national nursing initiative.* London: DH, 2001.

11 Maryon Davis A, Giles A, Rona R. *Tackling obesity: a toolbox for local partnership action.* London: Faculty of Public Health Medicine of the Royal Colleges of Physicians of the UK, 2000.

8 | Education and training of doctors in nutrition

SUMMARY

▪ Nutrition should be promoted as essential for learning across the entire undergraduate medical curriculum, with teaching of nutrition drawing widely on skills across disciplines and professions.

▪ Postgraduate nutritional training should form a continuum and lead to an appreciation that nutrition is important to all disciplines of medicine.

▪ Doctors should ensure that they remain familiar with up-to-date information about nutritional health and should regard this as an essential element of their continuing professional development.

▪ Clinical teachers should be encouraged to attend multiprofessional courses on nutrition in order to extend their knowledge and expertise.

▪ The Royal College of Physicians will build on its capacity to teach, contribute to public debate and influence national policy on nutrition.

8.1 Introduction

Nutrition forms part of every medical discipline. Medical curricula contain a wealth of information relevant to diet and nutrition, but generally represent a classical approach through biochemistry and physiology. It remains uncommon for nutrition to be taught as metabolism at the whole body level which would enable doctors to understand how function is maintained in health and disturbed by disease. The need for improved medical undergraduate training in nutrition was the subject of a report in 1983 by a task force of the British Nutrition Foundation.[1] Partly as a result of this, academic departments of human nutrition were established in some medical schools. A start has been made in devising and providing an integrated course in clinical nutrition for undergraduates,[2] and a working group of academic nutritionists, the Stratford Executive Group, estimated that about half of the UK medical schools would include a specific course on human nutrition after 1996.[3] However, it is generally acknowledged that many recently trained doctors still have an inadequate knowledge of the nutritional aspects of health promotion and disease treatment.

8.2 The core curriculum for nutrition

The need for better training in human nutrition is now recognised in all disciplines of health care. In 1994, the Government's Nutrition Task Force, created under the Health of the Nation initiative, published *A core curriculum for nutrition in the education of health professionals.*[4] This identifies a minimum core of essential knowledge for all health professionals. The curriculum was designed, among other aims, to enable all health professionals including doctors, to:

- appreciate the importance and relevance of nutrition to the promotion of good health and the prevention and treatment of disease
- describe the basic scientific principles of human nutrition
- identify nutrition-related problems in individuals and the community
- give consistent and sound dietary advice
- provide appropriate and safe clinical nutritional support, and know how and when to refer to a state-registered dietitian or another specialist in clinical nutrition.

There are few doctors recognised as specialists in clinical nutrition because there is no recognised pathway or accreditation programme in 'clinical nutrition' embedded within any major specialty.

The curriculum was divided into three sections, the first two of which should be covered for doctors during undergraduate training (but this cannot be taken for granted):

- *Principles of nutritional science* – includes foods and nutrients, metabolic processes, physical activity, effect of diet and nutrient status on biochemistry and organ function
- *Public health nutrition* – includes the average diet, lifestyle and risk factors, dietary reference values, nutritional surveillance, education and motivation, food policies and composition.

The third – *clinical nutrition and nutritional support* – provides a useful focus for the College in both General Professional and Higher (specialist) Training since it covers:

- assessment of clinical and functional metabolic state, effect of functional state on nutritional intake and status, and effect of status on clinical outcomes
- anorexia and starvation, response to injury, and infection and stress
- altered nutritional requirements in relevant disease states, unusual requirements

▪ general principles of nutritional support, routes of support
▪ basis of nutrition-related diseases, therapeutic diets, weight reduction
▪ drug–nutrient interactions.

8.3 Current situation in undergraduate medical training

There have been advances in teaching nutrition to medical students since the publication of *Nutrition for medical students.*[3] However, the time allocated to nutritional issues remains difficult to identify, and information about how well nutrition is incorporated into curricula using problem-based learning as the core method of medical education is not available. This deficiency of information is particularly disappointing for the following reasons:

▪ Human nutrition can be incorporated as an integrated theme: it can link basic sciences, clinical and public health aspects of health and disease in the core curriculum throughout the period of study, and should be included as part of a patient's clinical assessment.

▪ Nutrition offers the potential of 'horizontal integration' across disciplines as a component of problem-based approaches.

▪ Nutrition is well suited to special study modules, particularly for public health nutrition.

▪ The assessment of knowledge and skills in human nutrition are well suited for assessment in an undergraduate Objective Structured Clinical Examination (OSCE).

8.4 Doctors in training

Current situation in General Professional Training (GPT)

The third edition of *A core curriculum for senior house officers*[5] includes the following sections on clinical nutrition in its general section on skills:

▪ assessment of nutritional state and its effect on clinical outcomes
▪ nutritional requirements in illness and the metabolic effect of injury and infection
▪ general principles of nutritional support and routes of support
▪ principles of the dietetic management of nutrition-related disorders.

Despite this initiative, nutrition is not regularly or systematically examined in the examinations of the Royal Medical Colleges including MRCP(UK).

The revised curriculum for general (internal) medicine will include nutrition. It draws attention to the nutritional component of disease and the importance of appropriate nutritional intervention to improve clinical well-being and outcome. It lists the following competencies in diagnosis and management:

▪ undernutrition – identification of underlying factors and their management

▪ overweight and obesity – identification and management of patients requiring weight reduction

▪ nutritional risk states – competencies in the recognition of sub-optimal nutrition that may contribute to risk of ill health

▪ general principles of nutritional support and the management of starvation.

8.5 Areas of good practice

There are many local examples of good nutritional practice within the UK. These include the establishment of nutrition support teams for both adults and children in some hospitals, structured clinics for diabetes care, and the establishment of specialist clinics for the management of obesity and hyperlipidaemia. The specialist and core skills that need strengthening in clinical training have been listed in *Specialist registrar training in clinical nutritional support*,[6] a report prepared for the Royal College of Physicians Committee on Gastroenterology. This has formed the basis for the new section on nutrition support in the JCHMT revised gastroenterology curriculum.

The guidance on the management of overweight and obese patients with particular reference to drugs, published by the College in December 1998, is an example of how the College has contributed to the knowledge about the treatment of nutritional disorders.[7] The establishment of a specific committee on nutrition by the College confirms the importance it ascribes to nutrition within medicine; the committee also is contributing to knowledge by the organisation of conferences concerned with nutrition.

In 1996, an intercollegiate group on nutrition was established and this now has representatives from 11 of the UK medical Royal Colleges, including the three Royal Colleges of Physicians. The group has established a course for doctors that focuses on the general principles of human nutrition, and is now developing courses that will be specifically orientated towards specialist training in nutrition related to clinical practice.

8.6 Recommendations

Nutrition remains poorly covered within physicians' training programmes. This needs to be urgently addressed in recognition of the importance of dietary factors in disease, and the predicted long-term outcome in a population that is living to a greater age, with attendant ill health and nutritional vulnerability, and becoming increasingly overweight and obese. The medical profession should therefore take a lead by ensuring that nutrition becomes an integral part of medical undergraduate, general professional and specialty training; training in nutrition should include both therapy of the sick patient (clinical nutrition) and the identification of nutrition as a determinant of risk for ill health.

Undergraduate medical education

All medical practitioners should have a basic level of competence in nutrition, integrated with and applied to other clinical knowledge. Teaching of nutrition should draw widely on available skills across disciplines and health professionals, including dietitians and nursing.

- Nutrition should be promoted as a model subject for teaching across the entire undergraduate medical curriculum, and the nutrition being taught should be relevant.
- Nutritional screening and assessment should be included as part of the teaching of clinical skills, and students should be instructed about relevant practical skills such as the assessment of swallowing.
- Nutritional topics should be assessed at all levels throughout undergraduate training – the OSCE provides a practical examination format.
- An agreed procedure for clinical assessment of the nutritional status of patients should be included as a core skill: this should be part of any routine examination.

The progress of medical schools in achieving these recommendations could be monitored by the Education Committee of the General Medical Council.

Doctors in training – General Professional and Specialist Training

The following steps should be taken to promote education in clinical nutrition during General Professional and Specialist Training.

Postgraduate nutritional training should form a continuum with undergraduate training and lead to an appreciation that nutrition is important in all disciplines of medicine. Doctors in training should be motivated to regard nutrition as important in the prevention and management of disease.

The Royal Colleges should make nutrition a discrete section within the core curricula documents and emphasise to senior house officers (SHOs) the importance of identifying risk from poor nutrition as well as the existence of disease. Nutrition should also feature within the record of in-training assessment (RITA) for specialist registrars.

- As part of the history and physical examination of every new patient, a written statement should always be made in the clinical notes about his/her nutritional state, and doctors should be aware of the influence of nutritional status on susceptibility to illness.

- Regular teaching sessions on nutrition should be included as part of SHO and specialist registrar training programmes – this should include guidance on nutritional assessment and nutritional requirements in health and disease and an appreciation of nutrition as a determinant of risk.

- Every specialty should include an appropriate reference to nutrition in their core curriculum.

- Clinical teachers should be encouraged to attend courses on nutrition such as that provided by the intercollegiate group.

- Questions on nutrition should be included in examinations for higher qualifications. Inclusion of questions on nutrition in professional examinations and incorporation into assessment procedures are the key to the acceptance of nutrition by teachers and students as an important and valued subject area.

It is suggested that the postgraduate deanery and the medical Royal Colleges monitor the achievement of these recommendations.

Doctors

The following recommendations for doctors are adapted from the recommendations for health professionals included in the *Core curriculum for nutrition*:[4]

- *Educational* – doctors are seen by the public as providers of authoritative information and advice on food, health and nutrition. Doctors should ensure that they remain familiar with up-to-date information about nutritional health. This should be regarded as an essential element of their continuing professional development.

- *Advisory* – doctors can influence food and nutrition policy in their own hospital setting and within the local community. They should be encouraged to nominate a lead for nutrition within every NHS trust and, where appropriate, be involved in nutrition management and the nutrition team. Job plans should reflect the importance of nutrition as a part of weekly duties.

- *Organisational* – doctors should be encouraged to initiate or contribute to programmes on nutrition by working either as individuals, through professional societies or other health care organisations. Training must include the management of this kind of work.

- *Investigatory* – doctors should be encouraged to consider research into nutritional topics as part of their work. This should include both applied basic and molecular science as well as clinical investigations. The government should acknowledge the importance of such research for nutrition through the provision of research funding.

Joint training for health professionals is desirable and the nutrition components for continuing professional training should be planned on a multidisciplinary basis wherever possible. The Royal Colleges should monitor the achievement of these recommendations through continuing professional development programmes. NHS trusts should also monitor the involvement of doctors in nutrition as part of clinical governance.

Royal College of Physicians

- The Royal College of Physicians should seek to build on its capacity to teach, contribute to public debate and influence national policy on nutrition by:
  - Recognising and bringing together those among its number with special interest in the various aspects of human nutrition.
  - Encouraging the development of knowledge about nutrition by those in higher (specialist) training and by established consultants – each specialty committee should review the need for nutritional expertise within its training programmes.
  - Acknowledging the importance of multiprofessional involvement for the provision of effective nutritional care, and encouraging close collaboration between medical and allied health care professionals.

- The Royal Colleges should consider making the management of clinical nutritional problems a recognised subspecialty of an associated major specialty (eg gastroenterology, diabetes and endocrinology, nephrology etc). A useful model is the subspecialty training for metabolic medicine that is part of chemical pathology specialist training; this is also available to the small number of trainees who are undertaking training in general (internal) medicine alone.

The Royal College of Physicians should contribute advice on standards of nutritional care in relation to clinical governance, as well as implications for public health. This report is an example of how the College may make a contribution to improving the standard of a patient's nutritional care.

References

1   British Nutrition Foundation. *Nutrition in medical education. Report of the British nutrition task force on human nutrition.* London: British Nutrition Foundation, 1983.

2   Powell-Tuck J, Summerbell C, Holsgrove G, Garrow J. Four years' experience of an undergraduate medical nutrition course. *J Roy Soc Med* 1997; **90**: 67–72.

3   Department of Health. *Nutrition for medical students: nutrition in the undergraduate medical curriculum.* In *Health of the nation* series. London: DH, 1995.

4   Department of Health. *Nutrition: core curriculum for nutrition in the education of health professionals.* In *Health of the nation* series. London: DH, 1994.

5   Royal College of Physicians. *A core curriculum for senior house officers.* London: RCP, 2001.

6   Royal College of Physicians. *Specialist registrar training in clinical nutritional support.* A report prepared for the RCP Committee on Gastroenterology. Unpublished.

7   Royal College of Physicians. *Clinical management of overweight and obese patients with particular reference to the use of drugs.* Report of a working party. London: RCP, 1998.

Appendix 1 – Members of the working party

Professor PG Kopelman MD, FRCP (Chair)
Professor of Clinical Medicine, Deputy Warden, Barts and The London, Queen Mary's School of Medicine and Dentistry, University of London

Emeritus Professor JE Lennard-Jones MD, DSc(Hon), FRCP, FRCS (Secretary)
Emeritus Professor of Gastroenterology, University of London; Emeritus Consultant Gastroenterologist, St. Mark's Hospital, London

Professor Sir George Alberti FRCP(Edin), FRCPath
President, Royal College of Physicians

Professor SP Allison MD, FRCP
Consultant Physician, Professor in Clinical Nutrition; Director, Clinical Nutrition Unit, University Hospital, Queen's Medical Centre, Nottingham

Dr SA Bruce MD, FRCP
Consultant Physician, Conquest Hospital, St Leonards-on-Sea; Chairman, British Geriatrics Society Gastroenterology and Nutrition Special Interest Group

Dr WR Burnham MA, MD, FRCP
Consultant Physician & Gastroenterologist, Chairman, Nutritional Advisory Group, Oldchurch Hospital, Romford

Mr GL Carlson Bsc, MD, FRCS
Consultant Surgeon, Hope Hospital, Salford; Chairman, Clinical Governance Committee, British Association for Parenteral and Enteral Nutrition

Mrs H Davidson BSc
Senior Dietitian, Queen's Medical Centre, Nottingham

Professor JSA Edwards PhD
Professor of Food Service, Worshipful Company of Cooks Centre for Culinary Research, Bournemouth University

Professor M Elia MB, ChB, BSc Hons, MD, FRCP
Professor of Clinical Nutrition & Metabolism and Honorary Consultant Physician, Institute of Human Nutrition, Southampton General Hospital

Professor Ian T Gilmore MD, FRCP
Registrar, Royal College of Physicians

Dr LV Jackson BSc, MRCGP, DCH, DFFP, Dip. Ther.
Branch Head, Nutrition Division, Food Standards Agency

Dr A Maryon Davis MB, Bchir, MSc, MRCP(UK)
Consultant and Senior Lecturer in Public Health Medicine, Lambeth, Southwark and Lewisham Health Authority and King's College, London

Mrs J McGovern BSc(Hons), RGN
Clinical Nurse Specialist in Nutrition on behalf of the National Nurses Nutrition Group

Dr DBA Silk MD, FRCP
Consultant Physician, Central Middlesex Hospital, London

Dr S Reddy MSc, PhD
Principal Nutritionist, Department of Health

Dr S Robinson MD, FRCP
Consultant Physician, St Mary's Hospital, London

Dr C Waine OBE, FRCGP, FRCPath
Director of External Relations, Sunderland Health Authority

Mr R Wilson BSc, SRD
Director of Nutrition and Dietetics, King's College Hospital, London

Appendix 2 – Selected reports

Audit Commission
Audit Commission, 1 Vincent Square, London SW1P 2PN
Acute hospital portfolio. Catering (2001)

British Association for Parenteral and Enteral Nutrition
BAPEN Office, Secure Hold Business Centre,
Studley Road, Redditch, Worcs BN98 7LG
Organisation of nutritional support in hospitals (1994)
Standards and guidelines for nutritional support of patients in hospitals
(1996)
Hospital food as treatment (2000)
Ethical and legal aspects of clinical hydration and nutritional support
(1998)
Guidelines for detection and management of malnutrition (2000)
Trends in artificial nutrition support in the UK during 1996-2000 (2001)

Council of Europe
Food and nutritional care in hospitals: how to prevent undernutrition.
Report and guidelines. Provisional edition, Partial Agreement in the
Social and Public Health Field (P-SG 9 2001) 11

Department of Health
The NHS Plan: a plan for investment: a plan for reform. Cm 4818 (2000)
National Service Framework for Coronary Heart Disease (2000)
National Service Framework for Older People (2001)
The essence of care: patient-focussed benchmarking for health care practitioners
(2001)

**Faculty of Public Health Medicine of the Royal Colleges of Physicians
of the United Kingdom**
4 St Andrews Place, London NW1 4LB
Tackling obesity: a toolbox for local partnership action (2000)

Health of the Nation Task Force
Department of Health
Nutrition and health. A management handbook (1994)
*Nutrition: core curriculum for nutrition in the education of health
professionals* (1994)
The contribution of state registered dietitians (1994)
Nutrition guidelines for hospital catering (1995)

Nutrition for medical student: nutrition in the undergraduate medical curriculum (1996)
Nutrition guidelines: a checklist for audit (1996)

National Audit Office
Tackling obesity in England (2001). London: The Stationery Office

NHS Executive
Hospital catering: delivering a quality service (1996)

Nuffield Trust
59 New Cavendish Street, London W1M 7RD
Managing nutrition in hospital: a recipe for quality (1999)

Royal College of Physicians of London
11 St Andrews Place, London, NW1 4LE
Overweight and obese patients: principles of management with particular reference to the use of drugs (1998, to be revised 2002)
Osteoporosis: clinical guidelines for prevention and treatment (1999)
Osteoporosis: clinical guidelines for prevention and treatment: update on pharmacological interventions and an algorithm for management (2000)
Medical treatment at the end of life: a position statement. *Clinical medicine*, 2001:**1**:115–17

Royal College of Psychiatrists
17 Belgrave Square, London SW1X 8PG
Eating disorders in the UK: policies for service development and training. Council report CR87 (2000)

University of Newcastle
The Centre For Health Services Research, University of Newcastle upon Tyne, 21 Claremont Place, Newcastle upon Tyne NE2 4AA
Eating Matters (1997)

Appendix 3 – Useful websites

Societies
The Nutrition Society: www.nutsoc.org.uk
British Association of Parenteral and Enteral Nutrition:
www.bapen.org.uk
European Society of Parenteral and Enteral Nutrition: www.espen.org
British Dietetic Association: www.bda.uk.com
Association for the Study of Obesity: www.aso.org.uk

Government organisations, non-governmental organisations and research institutes
British Nutrition Foundation: www.nutrition.org.uk
Department of Health: www.doh.gov.uk
Food Standards Agency: www.food.gov.uk
Scientific Advisory Committee on Nutrition: www.sacn.gov.uk